The Ultimate Dash Diet Cookbook for Beginners

2000 Days of Quick, Easy, Delicious, and Budget-Friendly Low-Sodium Recipes to Lower Blood Pressure, Complete with a 30-Day Meal Plan, Grocery Lists, and a Personalized Health Journal for Lazy People

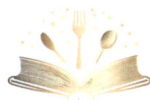

BiteBooks

Bite Books

Contents

BiteBooks is a USA-based culinary brand committed to producing high-quality cookbooks for food lovers of all levels. Each recipe is carefully crafted to ensure both ease and delicious results, making cooking an enjoyable experience. With a focus on quality and creativity, BiteBooks cookbooks are designed to inspire your culinary journey and bring people together through food. Explore new flavors, master classic dishes, and enjoy the process with BiteBooks, where every bite tells a story.

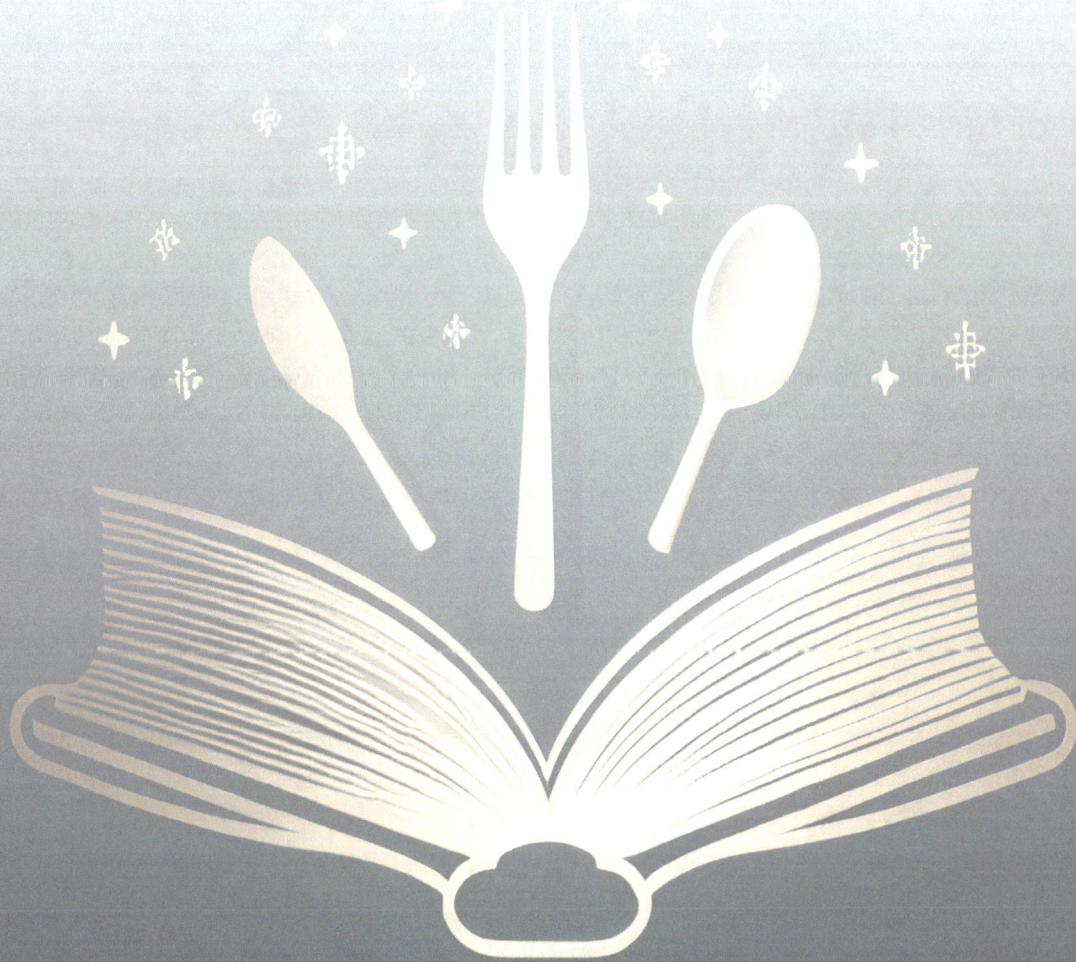

BiteBooks

Introduction

Welcome Message

Welcome to the DASH Diet Cookbook for Beginners! This comprehensive guide is designed to help you adopt a heart-healthy, balanced approach to eating that has been consistently ranked among the top diets for overall health and wellness. Whether your goal is to manage blood pressure, achieve sustainable weight loss, or enjoy a variety of nutritious meals, this cookbook is here to equip you with the knowledge and tools needed for success. Each section is carefully crafted with the beginner in mind, combining easy-to-follow recipes, structured meal plans, and practical advice to support your journey toward better health.

Overview of the DASH Diet

The DASH (Dietary Approaches to Stop Hypertension) diet is much more than just a temporary eating plan; it's a sustainable lifestyle supported by extensive clinical research and endorsed by leading health experts. Central to its approach is an emphasis on nutrient-rich foods, such as fruits, vegetables, lean proteins, whole grains, and low-fat dairy products. Key minerals like potassium, calcium, and magnesium are prioritized for their critical roles in reducing blood pressure and supporting cardiovascular health. Unlike restrictive diets, DASH encourages balance, promoting foods low in sodium and minimizing the intake of highly processed items, all while allowing room for personal taste preferences.

Benefits of a DASH Diet

Embracing the DASH diet can result in a multitude of health improvements, such as:

- **Lower Blood Pressure**: Multiple studies, including those supported by the National Heart, Lung, and Blood Institute (NHLBI), have demonstrated significant reductions in both systolic and diastolic blood pressure when adhering to the DASH plan.

- **Heart Disease Prevention:** With a focus on heart-healthy foods, the diet aids in lowering cholesterol and reducing the risk of cardiovascular conditions.

- **Weight Management**: The DASH diet's nutrient-dense, low-calorie food selection helps in achieving and maintaining a healthy weight without sacrificing flavor or satiety.

- **Enhanced Overall Wellness:** Balanced meals packed with vitamins, minerals, and fiber boost energy levels, enhance immune function, and contribute to long-term wellness.

How to Use This Book

This book is organized to provide clear, progressive guidance. It begins by establishing a solid foundation of knowledge about the DASH diet and advances into practical meal plans and diverse recipes sorted by meal type, including breakfast, lunch, dinner, sides, snacks, drinks, and desserts. A dedicated section on personal health journaling will help you track your progress, set realistic goals, and stay motivated. This cookbook is your roadmap to a seamless integration of the DASH diet into daily life, starting with manageable changes and gradually incorporating more advanced dietary habits.

Chapter 1: Getting Started with the DASH Diet

Introduction to the Principles of the DASH Diet

At the heart of the DASH diet lies the philosophy of balanced, minimally processed nutrition. It promotes:

- **Vegetables and Fruits:** A vital source of potassium and dietary fiber, these form the core of the diet and contribute to lowering blood pressure.

- **Whole Grains:** Nutrient-rich foods like brown rice, quinoa, and whole wheat bread help maintain energy levels and support digestive health.

- **Lean Proteins:** Options such as chicken, turkey, fish, and plant-based proteins like lentils and beans are encouraged.

- **Low-Fat Dairy:** These sources provide calcium, essential for maintaining strong bones and supporting heart health.

- **Healthy Fats:** Olive oil, nuts, and seeds contribute heart-friendly unsaturated fats that are integral to overall health.

The Science Behind the DASH Diet

The DASH diet has strong roots in science and medicine. Endorsed by organizations like the American Heart Association and Mayo Clinic, its efficacy is backed by numerous studies. The primary mechanism of the diet is its high intake of potassium-rich foods, which counteract sodium's effects and support healthy blood pressure. By focusing on whole foods, the diet naturally lowers sodium intake, which is a significant factor in managing hypertension. Research has shown that individuals adhering to the DASH diet can see a noticeable improvement in blood pressure and cardiovascular health in as little as two weeks.

Essential Kitchen Tools and Ingredients

A successful transition to the DASH diet starts with a well-equipped kitchen:

- **Basic Tools:** Ensure you have essentials like a cutting board, high-quality knives, measuring spoons, measuring cups, a food processor, a steamer, and a non-stick skillet.

- **Pantry Staples**: Stock up on olive oil, dried and canned beans, brown rice, quinoa, bulgur, low-sodium broth, a selection of herbs and spices, and a variety of nuts and seeds.

- **Fresh Produce:** Keep a supply of leafy greens, carrots, bell peppers, tomatoes, cucumbers, and seasonal fruits.

- **Proteins:** Include lean meats like chicken and turkey, as well as fish and legumes.

- **Dairy:** Opt for low-fat or non-fat milk, cheese, and yogurt.

Tips for Transitioning to a DASH Diet

Shifting to a new way of eating may seem daunting, but these tips can simplify the process:

- **Start Gradually:** Begin by substituting high-sodium snacks and processed foods with fresh fruits and raw vegetables.

- **Plan Your Meals:** Crafting a weekly meal plan takes the guesswork out of meal preparation and ensures you stay consistent.

- **Try New Recipes:** Experiment with a few new DASH-friendly recipes each week to diversify your meals and discover new favorites.

- **Stay Hydrated:** Drinking water and unsweetened herbal teas can help maintain hydration and keep sugar intake low.

- **Mindful Eating:** Focus on eating without distractions to better appreciate your meals and recognize fullness cues.

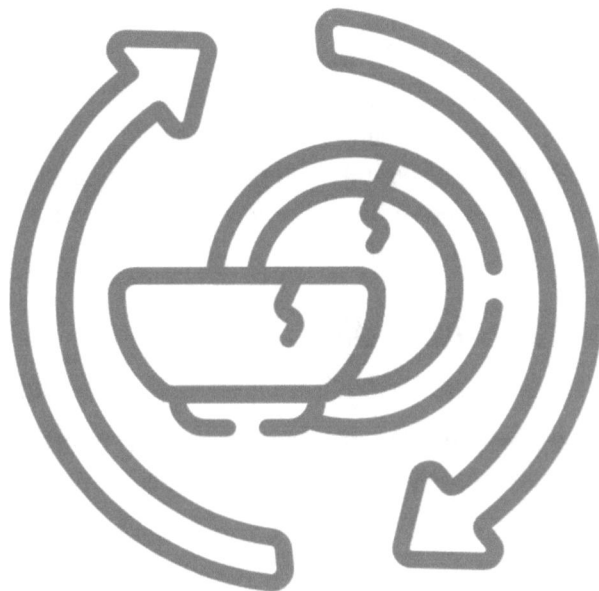

Chapter 2: 30-Day Meal Plan

Day	Breakfast	Lunch	Dinner
DAY 1	Oatmeal with Blueberries and Almonds, 16	Lentil and Veggie Salad, 27	Lemon Herb Chicken with Brown Rice, 38
DAY 2	Spinach and Mushroom Omelet, 16	Chicken Caesar Salad with Greek Yogurt Dressing, 27	Grilled Tilapia with Garlic and Lemon, 38
DAY 3	Greek Yogurt Parfait with Honey and Walnuts, 17	Grilled Shrimp Salad with, 28 Avocado	Herb-Crusted Pork Tenderloin, 40
DAY 4	Avocado Toast with Tomatoes and Basil, 17	Chickpea and Quinoa Salad, 28	Baked Cod with Cherry Tomatoes, 39
DAY 5	Banana Pancakes with Chia Seeds, 18	Turkey and Spinach Wraps, 29	Beef Stir-Fry with Broccoli, 39
DAY 6	Veggie Scramble with Bell Peppers, 18	Zucchini Noodles with Pesto, 29	Chicken and Vegetable Skewers, 40
DAY 7	Sweet Potato Breakfast Hash, 21	Tuna Salad with Lemon and Dill, 30	Mediterranean Chicken with Olives, 43
DAY 8	Whole Wheat Muffins with Berries, 19	Grilled Chicken and Mango Salad, 30	Baked Eggplant Parmesan, 41
DAY 9	Egg White Frittata with Spinach, 20	Kale Salad with Cranberries and Almonds, 31	Roasted Lamb with Rosemary and Thyme, 42
DAY 10	Quinoa Breakfast Bowl with Fruit, 20	Mediterranean Couscous Bowl, 31	Vegetable Stir-Fry with Tofu, 42

DAY 11	Smoked Salmon and Dill Bagel, 19	Cucumber and Hummus Sandwich, 22	Spaghetti Squash with Turkey Marinara, 43
DAY 12	Cottage Cheese with Pineapple and Mint, 21	Grilled Salmon Salad with Spinach, 34	Lemon Garlic Shrimp with Couscous, 44
DAY 13	Apple Cinnamon Overnight Oats, 22	Tomato Basil Soup with Grilled Cheese, 34	Honey Mustard Salmon, 44
DAY 14	Chia Seed Pudding with Mango, 22	Quinoa and Beet Salad, 35	Ratatouille with Fresh Basil, 45
DAY 15	Tomato and Avocado Egg Toast, 23	Caprese Salad with Balsamic Glaze, 35	Chicken Piccata with Capers, 46
DAY 16	Baked Oatmeal with Banana and Walnuts, 23	Soba Noodle Salad with Sesame Dressing, 36	Roasted Cauliflower Steaks, 46
DAY 17	Breakfast Smoothie with Spinach and Kiwi, 24	Tabbouleh with Grilled Chicken, 33	Grilled Mahi-Mahi with Mango Salsa, 47
DAY 18	Poached Egg with Asparagus, 24	Spicy Black Bean and Corn Salad, 33	Sweet Potato and Black Bean Enchiladas, 47
DAY 19	Baked Eggs in Avocado, 25	Chickpea Curry with Spinach, 36	Herb-Crusted Pork Tenderloin, 40
DAY 20	Savory Greek Yogurt Bowl with Cucumbers and Herbs, 25	Lentil and Veggie Salad, 27	Lemon Herb Chicken with Brown Rice, 38
DAY 21	Oatmeal with Blueberries and Almonds, 16	Grilled Shrimp Salad with Avocado, 28	Beef Stir-Fry with Broccoli, 39
DAY 22	Spinach and Mushroom Omelet, 16	Chicken Caesar Salad with Greek Yogurt Dressing, 27	Herb-Crusted Pork Tenderloin, 40
DAY 23	Greek Yogurt Parfait with Honey and Walnuts, 17	Chickpea and Quinoa Salad, 28	Roasted Lamb with Rosemary and Thyme, 42

DAY 24	Avocado Toast with Tomatoes and Basil, 17	Turkey and Spinach Wraps, 29	Baked Eggplant Parmesan, 41
DAY 25	Banana Pancakes with Chia Seeds, 18	Zucchini Noodles with Pesto, 29	Chicken and Vegetable Skewers, 40
DAY 26	Veggie Scramble with Bell Peppers, 18	Tuna Salad with Lemon and Dill, 30	Mediterranean Chicken with Olives, 43
DAY 27	Sweet Potato Breakfast Hash, 21	Grilled Chicken and Mango Salad, 30	Lemon Garlic Shrimp with Couscous, 44
DAY 28	Whole Wheat Muffins with Berries, 19	Kale Salad with Cranberries and Almonds, 31	Spaghetti Squash with Turkey Marinara, 43
DAY 29	Egg White Frittata with Spinach, 20	Mediterranean Couscous Bowl, 31	Vegetable Stir-Fry with Tofu, 42
DAY 30	Quinoa Breakfast Bowl with Fruit, 20	Tomato Basil Soup with Grilled Cheese, 34	Chicken Piccata with Capers, 46

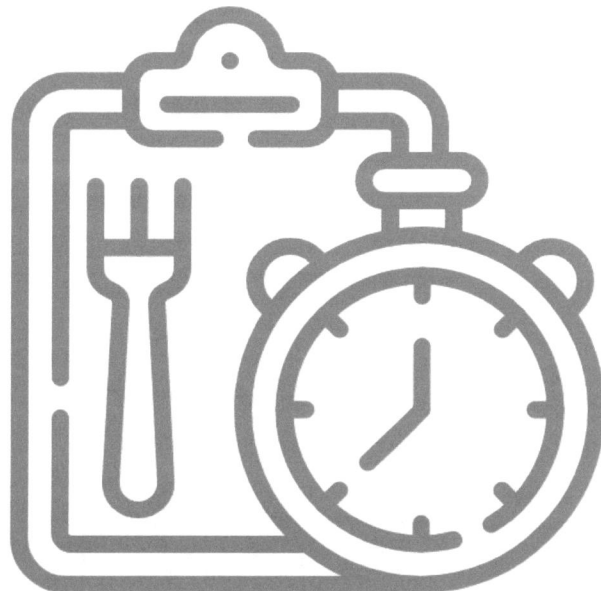

Grocery List for 30 Days

Produce:

- Leafy greens (e.g., spinach, kale, romaine lettuce): 10 lbs
- Asparagus: 1 bunch
- Green beans: 1 lb
- Brussels sprouts: 1 lb
- Red cabbage: 1/2 head
- Celery: 2 stalk
- Tomatoes: 20 large
- Bell peppers (mixed colors): 12
- Zucchini: 8 medium
- Sweet potatoes: 10 lbs
- Avocados: 15
- Carrots: 5 lbs
- Cucumbers: 6 large
- Broccoli: 5 lbs
- Cauliflower: 3 heads
- Bananas: 20
- Apples: 15
- Berries (strawberries, blueberries, mixed): 8 pints
- Grapes: 5 lbs
- Lemons: 10
- Limes: 5
- Oranges: 10
- Pineapple: 2 whole
- Mangoes: 4
- Fresh herbs (parsley, basil, mint, dill): 3 bunches each

Proteins:

- Lamb (leg or shoulder): 2 lbs
- Edamame: 2 cups (in pods)
- Chicken breast: 10 lbs
- Lean ground turkey: 8 lbs
- Salmon fillets: 6 lbs
- Smoked salmon: 6 oz
- Cod fillets: 4 lbs
- Shrimp: 3 lbs
- Pork tenderloin: 3 lbs
- Tilapia: 4 lbs
- Eggs: 3 dozen
- Tofu: 4 blocks
- Canned tuna: 6 cans
- Bison or lean ground beef: 4 lbs

Dairy:

- Heavy cream: 1 pint
- Cream cheese: 1/2 lb
- Greek yogurt (plain, low-fat): 4 tubs (32 oz each)
- Cottage cheese: 3 tubs (16 oz each)
- Low-fat milk or almond milk: 2 gallons
- Ricotta cheese: 2 containers (15 oz each)
- Low-fat cheese (cheddar, feta, parmesan): 3 lbs combined

Grains and Legumes:

- Whole wheat bread: 4 loaves
- Couscous: 2lbs
- Quinoa: 3 lbs
- Brown rice: 5 lbs
- Lentils: 2 lbs
- Chickpeas (canned or dried): 6 cans or 2 lbs dried
- Black beans (canned): 4 cans
- Oats: 3 lbs
- Whole wheat pasta: 2 lbs
- Bulgur: 3 lbs
- Soba noodles: 2 lbs
- Corn tortillas: 8

Snacks and Pantry Staples:

- Almonds: 2 lbs
- Chia seeds: 1 lb
- Peanut butter or almond butter: 2 jars (16 oz each)
- Dark chocolate squares: 2 packs
- Olive oil: 3 bottles (750 ml each)

- Balsamic vinegar: 1 bottle (16 oz)
- Low-sodium vegetable broth: 6 cartons (32 oz each)
- Canned tomatoes: 8 cans (14 oz each)
- Hummus: 2 tubs (16 oz each)
- Raisins: 1/4 cup
- Pine nuts: 1/4 cup
- Tahini: 1 small jar
- 2 Cups breadcrumbs

Spices and Seasonings:
- Garlic: 3 heads
- Ground cinnamon: 1 jar
- Paprika: 1 jar

- Cumin: 1 jar
- Black pepper: 1 jar
- Salt: 1 container
- Oregano: 1 jar
- Rosemary: 1 jar
- Thyme: 1 jar
- Dill: 1 jar
- Capers: 1 small jar
- Paprika: 1 jar (extra for recipes)
- Cumin: 1 jar (extra for recipes)
- Cinnamon: 1 jar (for dessert and Moroccan carrots)

Meal Prep Tips for DASH Diet Success

1. Start Small and Build Momentum

Transitioning to a new way of eating can be overwhelming, so start by prepping a few meals or snacks for the week. Gradually increase the number as you get comfortable. For example:

- Begin with breakfast prep (overnight oats, fruit bowls).

- Add lunch options like salads or wraps in the second week.

- Move on to prepping complete dinners.

2. Focus on Versatile Ingredients

Choose ingredients that can be used in multiple recipes to save time and reduce waste:

- Proteins: Cook a batch of grilled chicken or turkey breast for salads, wraps, and dinners.

- Whole Grains: Prepare quinoa, brown rice, or bulgur for grain bowls, side dishes, or stir-fries.

- Vegetables: Roast a tray of mixed vegetables (carrots, broccoli, zucchini) to use in salads, bowls, or as snacks.

3. Prep Snacks in Advance

Having DASH-friendly snacks ready can help curb unhealthy cravings. Some ideas include:

- Cut-up vegetables like carrots, celery, and bell peppers with hummus or Greek yogurt dip.

- Pre-portion unsalted nuts or seeds into small containers.

- Prepare fruit salads or slice fresh fruit for quick grabs.

4. Use Time-Saving Tools

Invest in kitchen gadgets that make meal prep faster and easier:

- Slow Cooker or Instant Pot: Great for soups, stews, and grains.

- Food Processor: Ideal for chopping veggies, making hummus, or preparing sauces.

- Reusable Containers: Use BPA-free containers for portioning meals and snacks.

5. Customize the Meal Plan

While the meal plan provides structure, make it work for your tastes and lifestyle:

- Swap ingredients you don't like with DASH-friendly alternatives (e.g., swap spinach for kale).

- Adjust portion sizes based on your energy needs or goals.

6. Batch Cook Essentials

Prepare large batches of staples that can be used throughout the week:

- Proteins: Grilled chicken, turkey meatballs, or boiled eggs.

- Whole Grains: Cook enough quinoa, brown rice, or couscous for several meals.

- Soups and Stews: Freeze single portions for easy lunches or dinners.

7. Label and Organize

Label containers with the meal name and date to avoid confusion and ensure freshness. Keep an organized fridge:

- Top shelf: Ready-to-eat meals.

- Middle shelf: Prepped ingredients.

- Bottom shelf: Raw proteins for cooking.

8. Keep Hydration in Mind

Prepare infused water jars with lemon, cucumber, or mint to encourage daily hydration. This supports the DASH diet's emphasis on reducing sugary beverages.

9. Simplify Grocery Shopping

To save time and avoid stress:

- Use the grocery list provided with your meal plan.

- Stick to the DASH-friendly sections of the store: fresh produce, lean meats, low-fat dairy, and whole grains.

- Shop for non-perishable staples like canned beans or olive oil in bulk.

10. Make It Fun

Involve your family or roommates in meal prep to share the workload. Turn on music, make it a challenge, or prepare meals together for bonding time.

11. Plan for Flexibility

Even with a solid plan, life happens. Keep a few emergency options ready, like:

- Pre-washed salad greens.

- Low-sodium canned soups or beans.

- Frozen vegetables or pre-cooked proteins.

12. Reflect and Adjust

At the end of each week:

- Note what worked well and what didn't.

- Adjust recipes or portion sizes to better fit your schedule, tastes, or health goals.

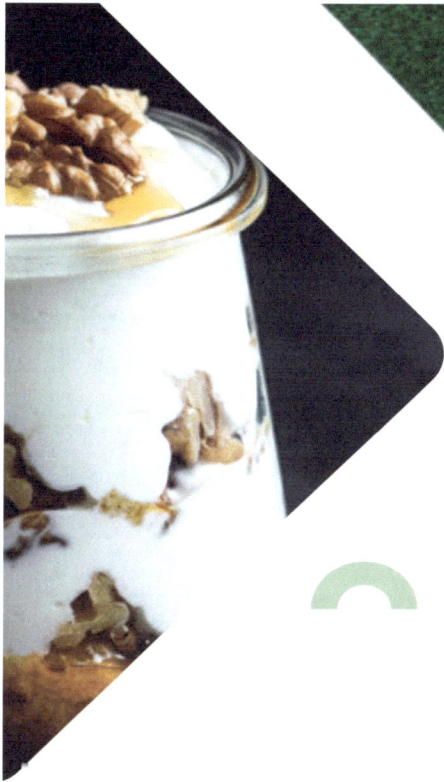

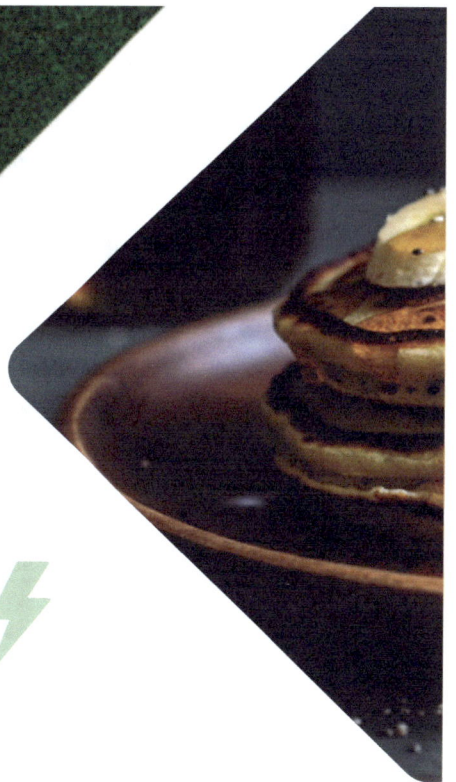

Chapter 3
Breakfast Recipes

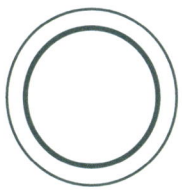

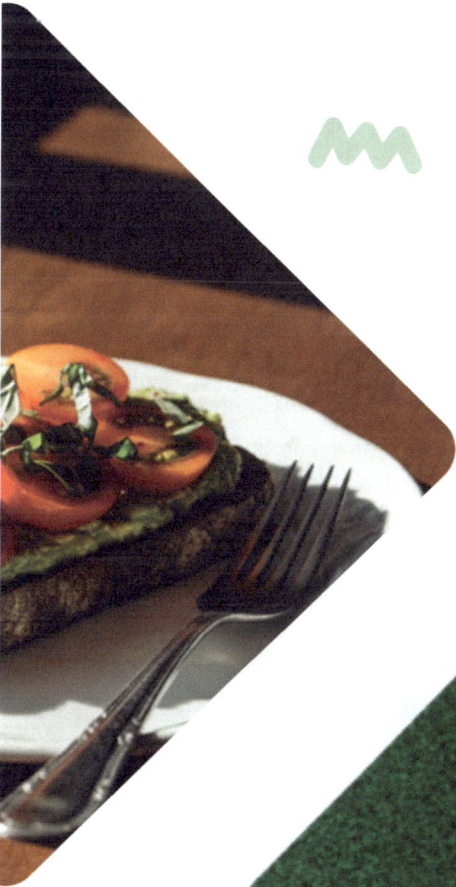

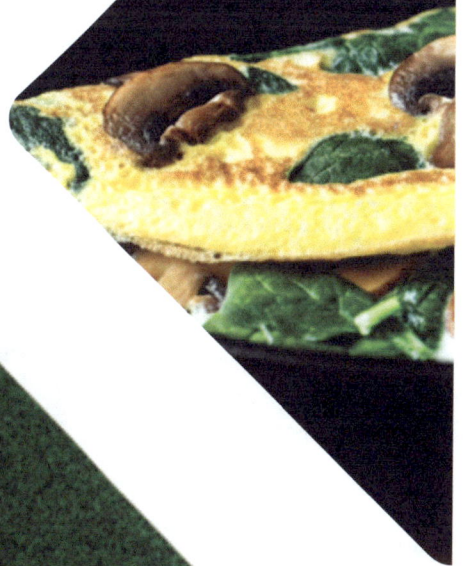

Oatmeal with Blueberries and Almonds

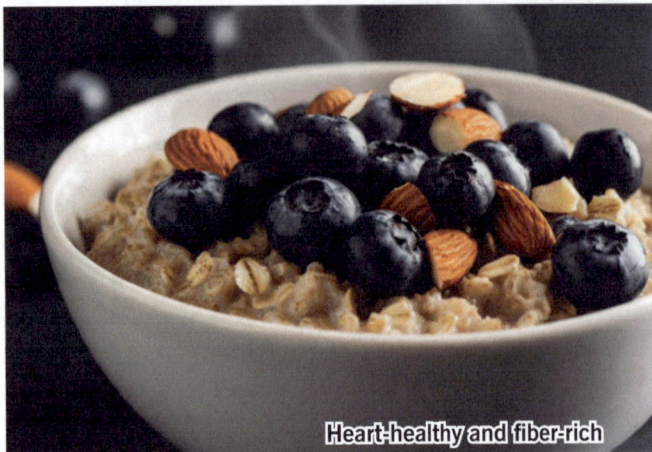

Heart-healthy and fiber-rich

2 servings

Prep Time **5** min

Cook Time **10** min

Nutritional
Calories: 280 kcal
Protein: 8g
Fats: 10g
Carbs: 45g

Instructions

1. In a medium saucepan, bring water or almond milk to a boil.
2. Add oats and a pinch of salt. Reduce heat to low and cook, stirring occasionally, for 5 minutes or until the oats reach your desired consistency.
3. Remove from heat and divide into two bowls.
4. Top with blueberries, sliced almonds, and a drizzle of honey if desired.
5. Serve warm.

Ingredients

- 1 cup rolled oats
- 2 cups water or almond milk
- 1/2 cup fresh blueberries
- 1/4 cup sliced almonds
- 1 tbsp honey (optional)
- A pinch of salt

Ingredient Availability

Available at major stores like Walmart, Target, Aldi, and Whole Foods.

Spinach and Mushroom Omelet

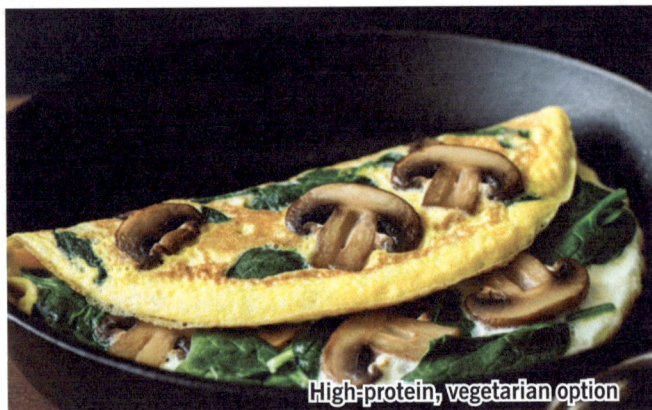

High-protein, vegetarian option

2 servings

Prep Time **5** min

Cook Time **10** min

Nutritional
Calories: 250 kcal
Protein: 18g
Fats: 17g
Carbs: 5g

Instructions

1. In a bowl, whisk eggs with milk, salt, and pepper.
2. Heat olive oil in a non-stick skillet over medium heat. Add mushrooms and sauté for 2 minutes.
3. Add spinach and cook until wilted, about 1 minute.
4. Pour egg mixture over the vegetables. Cook for 2-3 minutes or until the eggs start to set.
5. Sprinkle cheese on one half of the omelet and fold the other half over.
6. Cook for another minute or until the cheese is melted. Serve warm.

Ingredients

- 4 large eggs
- 1 cup fresh spinach, chopped
- 1/2 cup mushrooms, sliced
- 1/4 cup shredded cheddar cheese
- 2 tbsp milk
- 1 tbsp olive oil
- Salt and pepper to taste

Ingredient Availability

Available at Walmart, Publix, Aldi, and Whole Foods.

Greek Yogurt Parfait with Honey and Walnuts

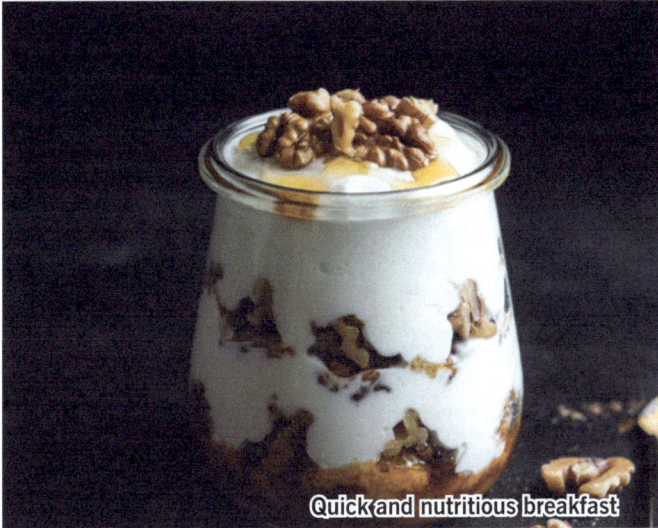

2 servings

Prep Time **5** min

Cook Time **0** min

Nutritional
Calories: 220 kcal
Protein: 10g
Fats: 12g
Carbs: 20g

Instructions

1. uctions:
2. Divide Greek yogurt into two serving glasses or bowls.
3. Layer with mixed berries and chopped walnuts.
4. Drizzle honey on top and serve immediately.

Quick and nutritious breakfast

Ingredients

- 1 cup Greek yogurt
- 2 tbsp honey
- 1/4 cup walnuts, chopped
- 1/2 cup mixed berries (e.g., strawberries, blueberries)

Ingredient Availability

Find all ingredients at stores like Target, Aldi, and Costco.

Avocado Toast with Tomatoes and Basil

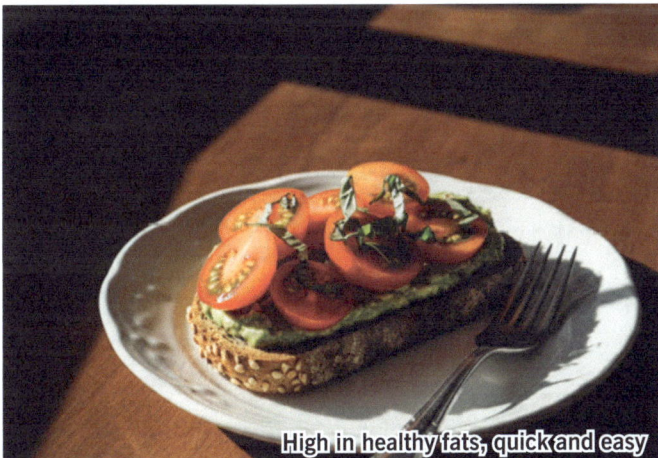

2 servings

Prep Time **10** min

Cook Time **0** min

Nutritional
Calories: 240 kcal
Protein: 5g
Fats: 15g
Carbs: 20g

Instructions

1. Toast the slices of whole-grain bread until golden and crispy.
2. Spread the mashed avocado evenly on each slice of toast.
3. Layer tomato slices over the avocado.
4. Add fresh basil leaves on top.
5. Drizzle with olive oil and season with salt and black pepper.
6. Serve immediately and enjoy.

High in healthy fats, quick and easy

Ingredients

- 2 slices whole-grain bread
- 1 ripe avocado, peeled and mashed
- 1 small tomato, thinly sliced
- 4–6 fresh basil leaves
- Salt and black pepper to taste
- 1 tbsp olive oil

Ingredient Availability

All ingredients can be found at Walmart, Publix, and Whole Foods.

Banana Pancakes with Chia Seeds

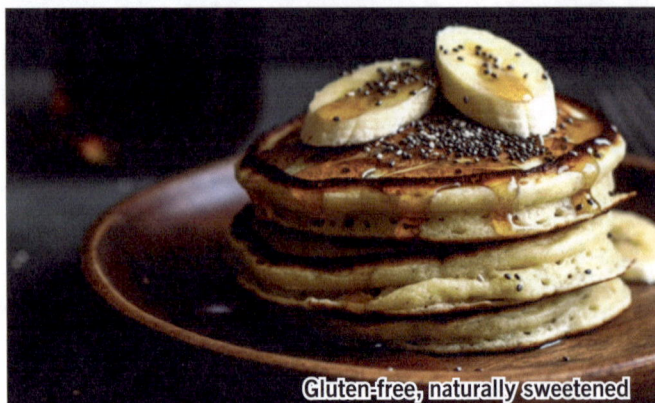

Gluten-free, naturally sweetened

🍴 4 servings

⏱ Prep Time **10** min

⏳ Cook Time **15** min

Nutritional
Calories: 180 kcal
Protein: 6g
Fats: 7g
Carbs: 25g

Ingredients

- 2 ripe bananas, mashed
- 2 large eggs
- 1/4 cup rolled oats
- 1 tbsp chia seeds
- 1/2 tsp baking powder
- 1/2 tsp cinnamon
- 1 tbsp coconut oil for cooking

Instructions

1. In a mixing bowl, combine the mashed bananas, eggs, rolled oats, chia seeds, baking powder, and cinnamon. Mix until a smooth batter forms.
2. Heat a non-stick skillet over medium heat and add coconut oil.
3. Spoon 1/4 cup of batter onto the skillet for each pancake.
4. Cook for 2–3 minutes on each side or until golden brown.
5. Serve warm, optionally topped with fresh banana slices or a drizzle of honey.

Ingredient Availability

Commonly available at Target, Aldi, and Whole Foods.

Veggie Scramble with Bell Peppers

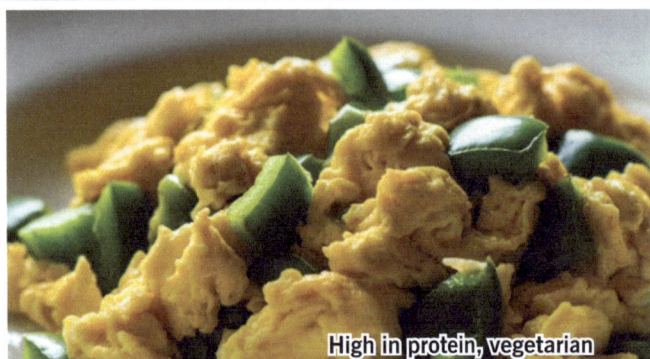

High in protein, vegetarian

🍴 2 servings

⏱ Prep Time **5** min

⏳ Cook Time **10** min

Nutritional
Calories: 190 kcal
Protein: 14g
Fats: 12g
Carbs: 6g

Ingredients

- 4 large eggs, beaten
- 1/2 red bell pepper, diced
- 1/2 green bell pepper, diced
- 1/4 cup red onion, chopped
- 2 tbsp low-fat milk
- Salt and black pepper to taste
- 1 tbsp olive oil
- Fresh parsley for garnish

Instructions

1. Heat olive oil in a skillet over medium heat.
2. Add the bell peppers and red onion, and sauté for 3–4 minutes until softened.
3. In a bowl, whisk the eggs with milk, salt, and pepper.
4. Pour the egg mixture into the skillet and scramble with the vegetables for 2–3 minutes or until cooked through.
5. Serve garnished with fresh parsley.

Ingredient Availability

Easily found at Aldi, Food Lion, and Harris Teeter.

Sweet Potato Breakfast Hash

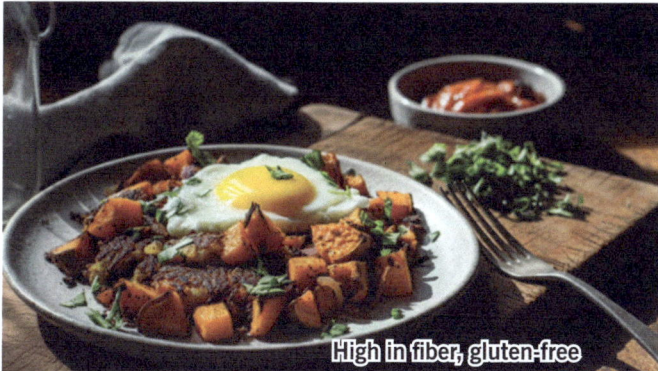

High in fiber, gluten-free

4 servings

Prep Time **10** min

Cook Time **20** min

Nutritional
Calories: 150 kcal
Protein: 3g
Fats: 8g
Carbs: 18g

Instructions

1. Preheat oven to 400°F (200°C).

2. In a bowl, toss sweet potatoes, onion, bell pepper, and garlic with olive oil, paprika, salt, and pepper.

3. Spread the mixture on a baking sheet and roast for 20 minutes or until the sweet potatoes are tender.

4. Serve warm, garnished with fresh parsley.

Ingredients

- 2 medium sweet potatoes, peeled and cubed
- 1 small red onion, diced
- 1 bell pepper (any color), diced
- 2 cloves garlic, minced
- 2 tbsp olive oil
- 1/2 tsp paprika
- Salt and black pepper to taste
- Fresh parsley for garnish

Ingredient Availability

Available at Walmart, Publix, and Whole Foods.

Whole Wheat Muffins with Berries

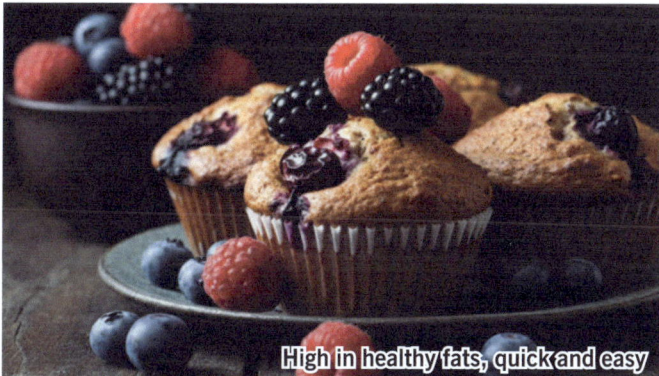

High in healthy fats, quick and easy

6 servings

Prep Time **10** min

Cook Time **20** min

Nutritional
Calories: 130 kcal
Protein: 4g
Fats: 2g
Carbs: 25g

Instructions

1. Preheat oven to 350°F (175°C) and line a muffin tin with paper liners.

2. In a bowl, mix the flour, baking powder, and salt.

3. In another bowl, combine the honey, applesauce, egg, and milk.

4. Gradually mix the dry ingredients into the wet ingredients until just combined. Fold in the berries.

5. Spoon the batter into the muffin tin and bake for 20 minutes or until a toothpick comes out clean.

6. Let cool before serving.

Ingredients

- 1 cup whole wheat flour
- 1/2 cup mixed berries (fresh or frozen)
- 1/4 cup honey
- 1/2 cup unsweetened applesauce
- 1/2 tsp baking powder
- 1/4 tsp salt
- 1 large egg, beaten
- 1/4 cup low-fat milk

Ingredient Availability

Available at Target, Costco, and Harris Teeter.

Egg White Frittata with Spinach

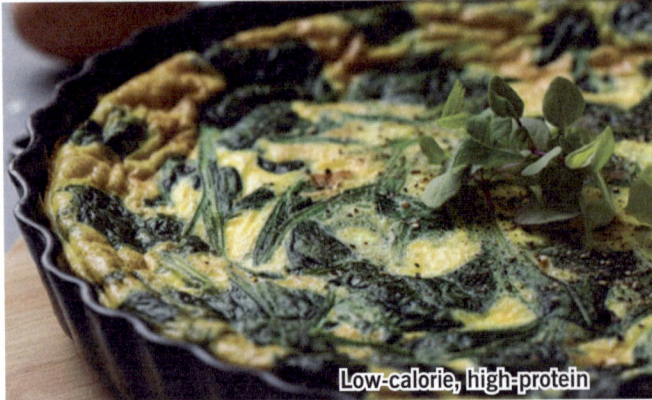

Low-calorie, high-protein

2 servings

Prep Time **5 min**

Cook Time **15 min**

Nutritional
Calories: 120 kcal
Protein: 16g
Fats: 6g
Carbs: 4g

Ingredients

- 6 large egg whites
- 1 cup fresh spinach, chopped
- 1/2 cup cherry tomatoes, halved
- 1/4 cup feta cheese, crumbled
- 1/2 tsp dried oregano
- Salt and black pepper to taste
- 1 tbsp olive oil

Instructions

1. Preheat the oven to 350°F (175°C).
2. Heat olive oil in an oven-safe skillet over medium heat. Add spinach and sauté until wilted, about 2 minutes.
3. Pour the egg whites over the spinach and arrange cherry tomatoes on top. Sprinkle with feta cheese, oregano, salt, and pepper.
4. Transfer the skillet to the oven and bake for 10–12 minutes or until the egg whites are set.
5. Serve warm and enjoy.

Ingredient Availability

All ingredients can be found at Walmart, Aldi, and Whole Foods.

Quinoa Breakfast Bowl with Fruit

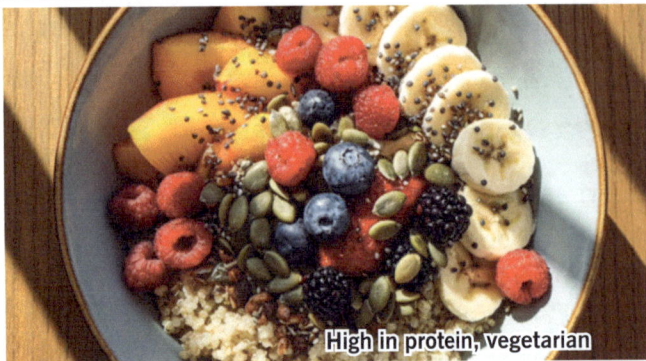

High in protein, vegetarian

2 servings

Prep Time **10 min**

Cook Time **15 min**

Nutritional
Calories: 250 kcal
Protein: 8g
Fats: 10g
Carbs: 35g

Ingredients

- 1/2 cup quinoa, rinsed
- 1 cup water
- 1/2 cup mixed berries (strawberries, blueberries, raspberries)
- 1 banana, sliced
- 2 tbsp almond butter
- 1 tbsp honey or maple syrup (optional)
- 1/4 tsp cinnamon

Instructions

1. Bring water to a boil in a small pot and add quinoa. Reduce heat and simmer for 15 minutes or until quinoa is cooked and water is absorbed.
2. Divide the quinoa into two bowls. Top each with mixed berries, banana slices, and a dollop of almond butter.
3. Drizzle with honey or maple syrup, if using, and sprinkle with cinnamon.
4. Serve warm or chilled.

Ingredient Availability

Found at Target, Publix, and Costco.

Smoked Salmon and Dill Bagel

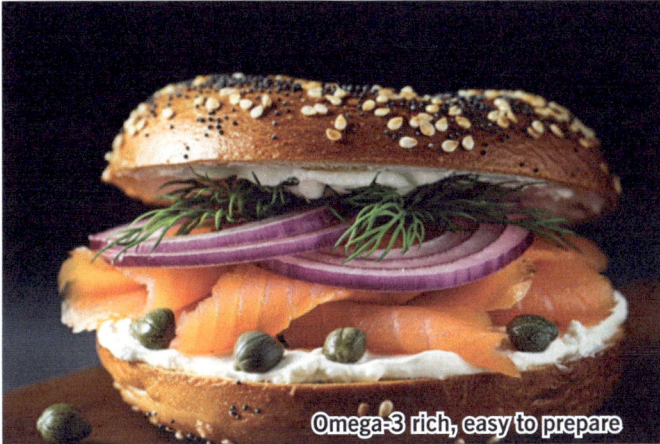

Omega-3 rich, easy to prepare

4 servings

Prep Time **5** min

Cook Time **0** min

Nutritional
Calories: 300 kcal
Protein: 15g
Fats: 12g
Carbs: 35g

Instructions

1. Toast the bagels until golden brown.
2. Spread cream cheese on each half of the bagel.
3. Layer smoked salmon over the cream cheese and sprinkle with dill.
4. Season with a little salt and black pepper. Serve with lemon slices for garnish.

Ingredients

- 2 whole-grain bagels, halved
- 4 oz smoked salmon
- 2 tbsp cream cheese
- 1 tbsp fresh dill, chopped
- 1/2 lemon, sliced for garnish
- Salt and black pepper to taste

Ingredient Availability

Available at Aldi, Harris Teeter, and Whole Foods.

Cottage Cheese with Pineapple and Mint

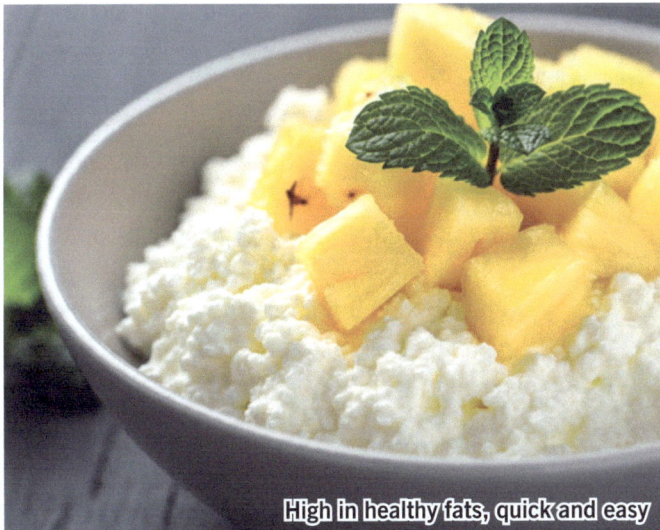

High in healthy fats, quick and easy

2 servings

Prep Time **5** min

Cook Time **0** min

Nutritional
Calories: 120 kcal
Protein: 15g
Fats: 2g
Carbs: 15g

Instructions

1. Divide cottage cheese between two bowls.
2. Top each with diced pineapple and sprinkle with fresh mint.
3. Drizzle with honey if desired.
4. Serve immediately.

Ingredients

- 1 cup low-fat cottage cheese
- 1/2 cup fresh pineapple, diced
- 1 tbsp fresh mint, chopped
- 1 tsp honey (optional)

Ingredient Availability

Commonly available at Walmart, Target, and Food Lion.

Apple Cinnamon Overnight Oats

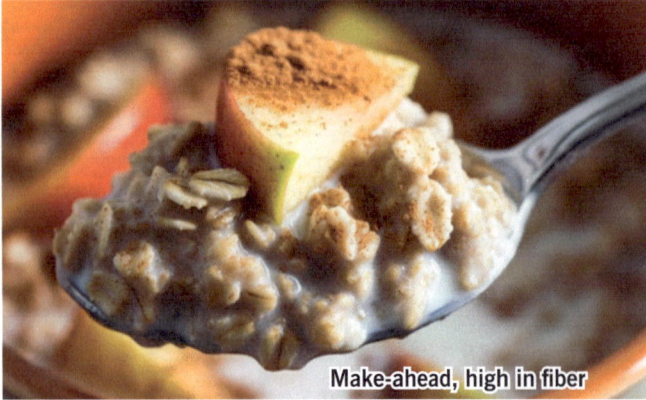

2 servings

Prep Time **5** min

Cook Time **0** min

Nutritional
Calories: 180 kcal
Protein: 6g
Fats: 4g
Carbs: 30g

Make-ahead, high in fiber

Instructions

1. In a mixing bowl, combine oats, almond milk, water, grated apple, cinnamon, and chia seeds.
2. Stir well and divide into two jars or bowls. Cover and refrigerate overnight.
3. In the morning, top with maple syrup if desired and serve chilled or at room temperature.

Ingredients

- 1 cup rolled oats
- 1/2 cup unsweetened almond milk
- 1/2 cup water
- 1 apple, peeled and grated
- 1/2 tsp cinnamon
- 1 tbsp chia seeds
- 1 tbsp maple syrup (optional)

Ingredient Availability

Available at Aldi, Publix, and Whole Foods.

Chia Seed Pudding with Mango

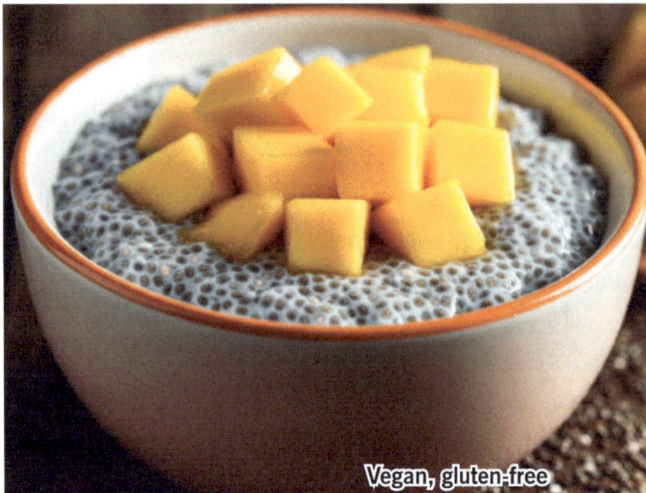

2 servings

Prep Time **5** min

Refrigeration **4** h

Nutritional
Calories: 220 kcal
Protein: 5g
Fats: 10g
Carbs: 30g

Vegan, gluten-free

Instructions

1. In a bowl, combine chia seeds, coconut milk, and vanilla extract. Stir well to prevent clumps.
2. Cover and refrigerate for at least 4 hours or overnight.
3. Divide the pudding into two serving bowls and top with diced mango and a drizzle of honey or maple syrup if desired.
4. Serve chilled.

Ingredients

- 1/4 cup chia seeds
- 1 cup coconut milk or almond milk
- 1 tbsp honey or maple syrup (optional)
- 1/2 cup mango, diced
- 1/2 tsp vanilla extract

Ingredient Availability

Found at Walmart, Target, and Whole Foods.

Tomato and Avocado Egg Toast

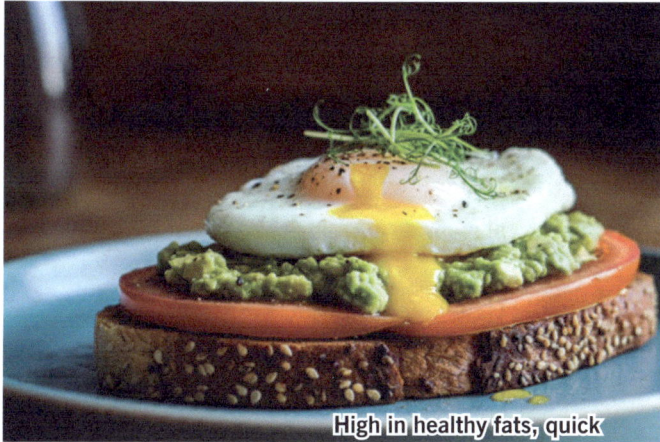

2 servings

Prep Time **5 min**

Cook Time **5 min**

Nutritional
Calories: 280 kcal
Protein: 12g
Fats: 18g
Carbs: 20g

Instructions

1. In a skillet, heat olive oil over medium heat and cook eggs sunny-side up or to desired doneness.

2. Top each slice of toasted bread with sliced avocado, tomato slices, and one cooked egg.

3. Season with salt and black pepper to taste.

4. Serve immediately.

High in healthy fats, quick

Ingredients

- 2 slices whole-grain bread, toasted
- 2 eggs
- 1 avocado, sliced
- 1 medium tomato, sliced
- Salt and black pepper to taste
- 1 tbsp olive oil

Ingredient Availability

Available at Aldi, Harris Teeter, and Publix.

Baked Oatmeal with Banana and Walnuts

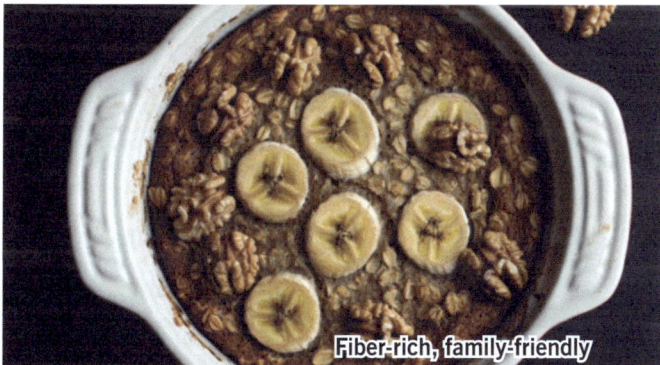

2 servings

Prep Time **10 min**

Cook Time **30 min**

Nutritional
Calories: 250 kcal
Protein: 6g
Fats: 10g
Carbs: 35g

Instructions

1. Preheat the oven to 350°F (175°C). Grease an 8x8-inch baking dish.

2. In a large bowl, combine rolled oats, walnuts, cinnamon, baking powder, and salt.

3. Stir in almond milk and honey or maple syrup until well mixed.

4. Pour the mixture into the prepared baking dish and top with banana slices.

5. Bake for 30 minutes or until golden brown. Let cool for a few minutes before serving.

Fiber-rich, family-friendly

Ingredients

- 2 cups rolled oats
- 1/2 cup walnuts, chopped
- 2 bananas, sliced
- 2 cups almond milk
- 1/4 cup honey or maple syrup
- 1 tsp cinnamon
- 1 tsp baking powder
- 1/2 tsp salt

Ingredient Availability

Found at Walmart, Costco, and Whole Foods.

Breakfast Smoothie with Spinach and Kiwi

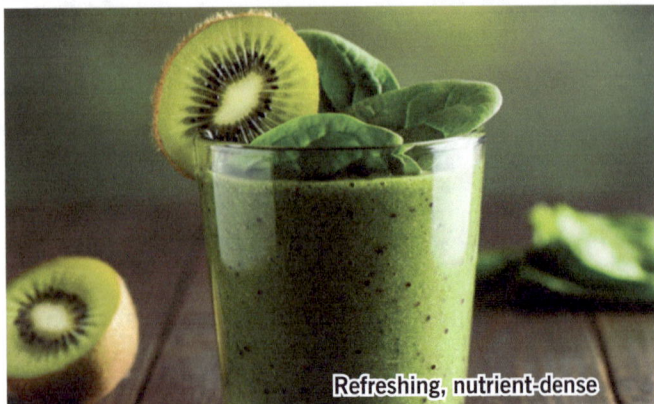
Refreshing, nutrient-dense

2 servings

Prep Time **5 min**

Cook Time **0 min**

Nutritional
Calories: 180 kcal
Protein: 8g
Fats: 2g
Carbs: 30g

Instructions

1. Combine all ingredients in a blender and blend until smooth.
2. Pour into glasses and serve immediately.

Ingredients

- 1 cup spinach, packed
- 2 kiwis, peeled and chopped
- 1 banana
- 1/2 cup Greek yogurt
- 1/2 cup water or almond milk
- 1 tbsp honey (optional)
- Ice cubes (optional)

Ingredient Availability

Available at Publix, Whole Foods, and Aldi.

Poached Egg with Asparagus

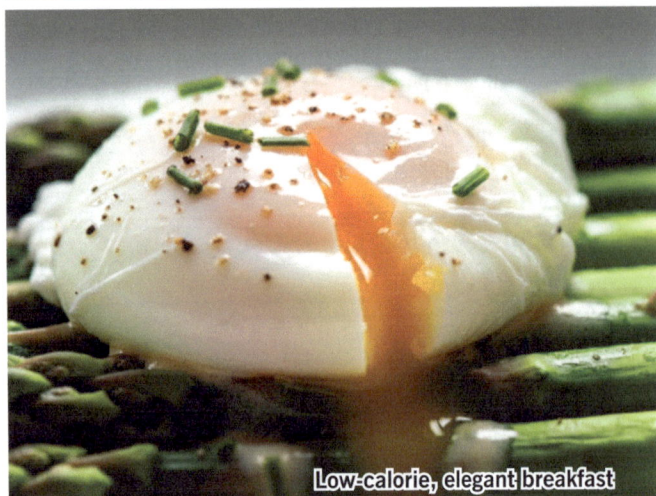
Low-calorie, elegant breakfast

2 servings

Prep Time **5 min**

Cook Time **10 min**

Nutritional
Calories: 150 kcal
Protein: 12g
Fats: 10g
Carbs: 4g

Instructions

1. Bring a pot of water with vinegar to a simmer. Crack each egg into a small bowl and gently slide it into the water. Poach for 3–4 minutes until whites are set.
2. Meanwhile, sauté asparagus in olive oil over medium heat for 5 minutes or until tender.
3. Serve poached eggs over sautéed asparagus and season with salt and black pepper.

Ingredients

- 4 eggs
- 1 bunch asparagus, trimmed
- 1 tbsp white vinegar
- Salt and black pepper to taste
- 1 tbsp olive oil

Ingredient Availability

Found at Harris Teeter, Aldi, and Costco.

Baked Eggs in Avocado

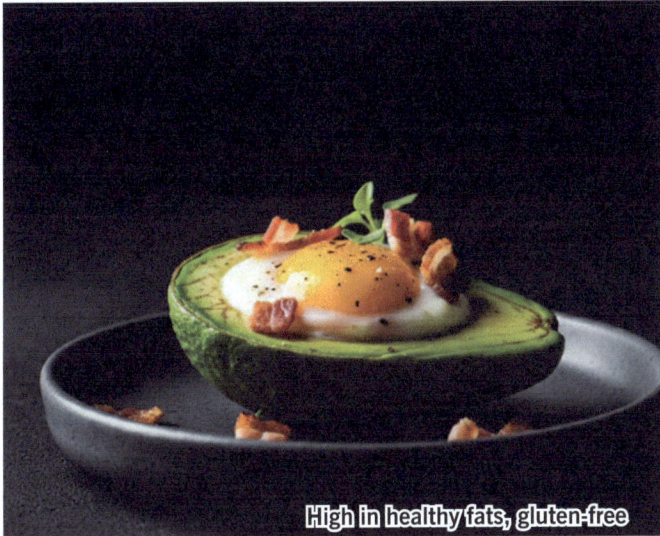

High in healthy fats, gluten-free

2 servings

Prep Time **5** min

Cook Time **15** min

Nutritional
Calories: 250 kcal
Protein: 10g
Fats: 20g
Carbs: 8g

Instructions

1. Preheat the oven to 425°F (220°C). Scoop out a bit of avocado flesh to make room for the eggs.
2. Place avocado halves in a baking dish and crack an egg into each.
3. Season with salt and pepper. Bake for 12–15 minutes or until the eggs are set.
4. Garnish with chives or parsley and serve warm.

Ingredients

- 2 avocados, halved and pitted
- 4 eggs
- Salt and black pepper to taste
- Fresh chives or parsley for garnish

Ingredient Availability

Available at Walmart, Target, and Whole Foods.

Savory Greek Yogurt Bowl with Cucumbers and Herbs

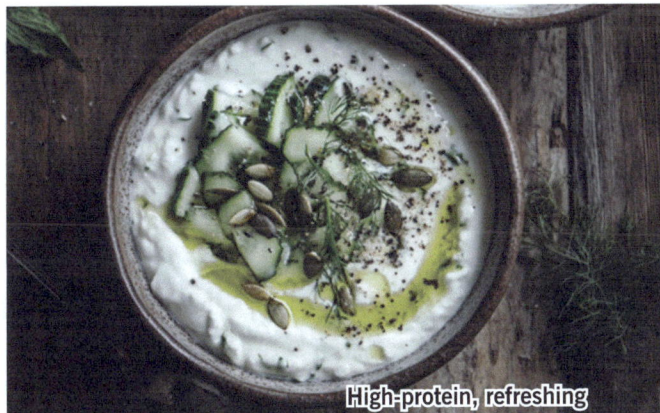

High-protein, refreshing

2 servings

Prep Time **5** min

Cook Time **0** min

Nutritional
Calories: 120 kcal
Protein: 15g
Fats: 5g
Carbs: 6g

Instructions

1. In a bowl, combine Greek yogurt, cucumber, dill, mint, and lemon zest. Mix until well blended.
2. Season with salt and black pepper.
3. Drizzle with olive oil before serving.

Ingredients

- 1 cup Greek yogurt
- 1/2 cucumber, diced
- 1 tbsp fresh dill, chopped
- 1 tbsp fresh mint, chopped
- 1 tsp lemon zest
- Salt and black pepper to taste
- Drizzle of olive oil

Ingredient Availability

Found at Publix, Aldi, and Whole Foods.

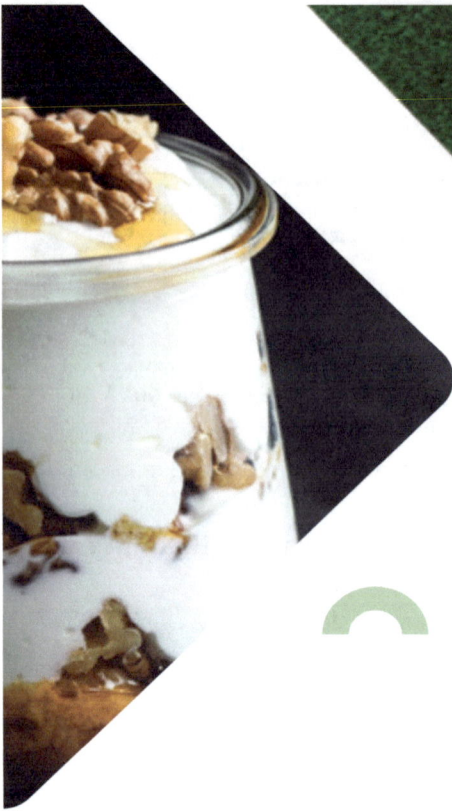

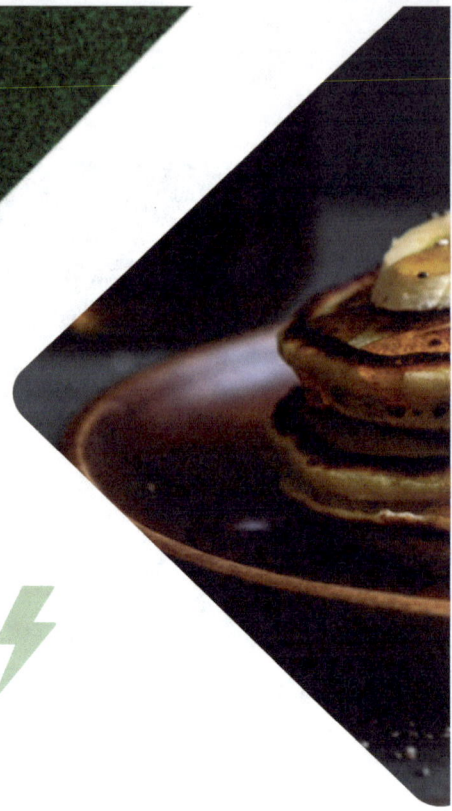

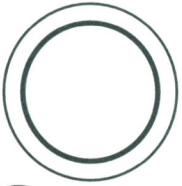

Chapter 4
Lunch Recipes

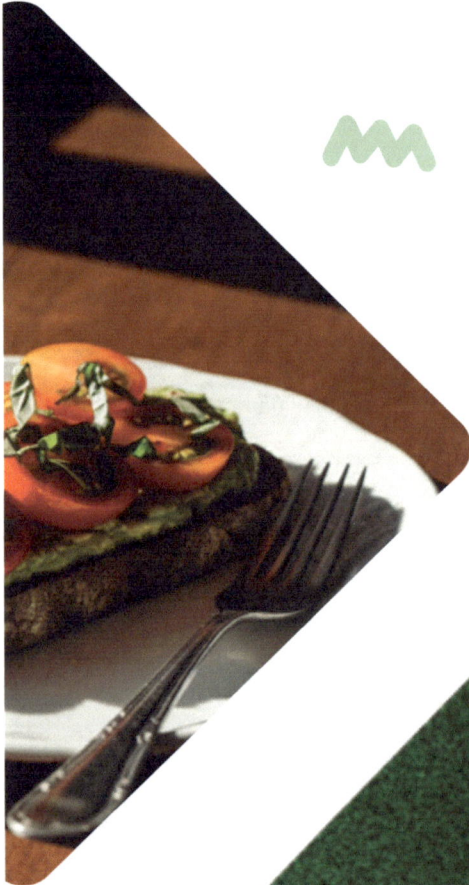

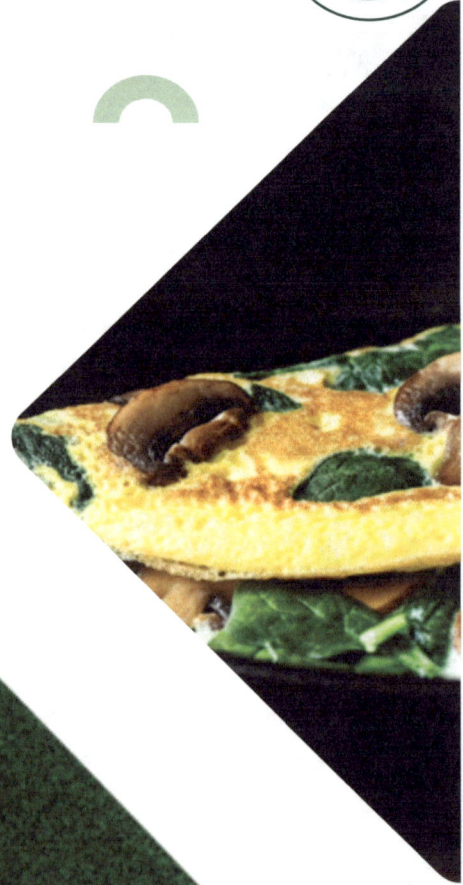

Lentil and Veggie Salad

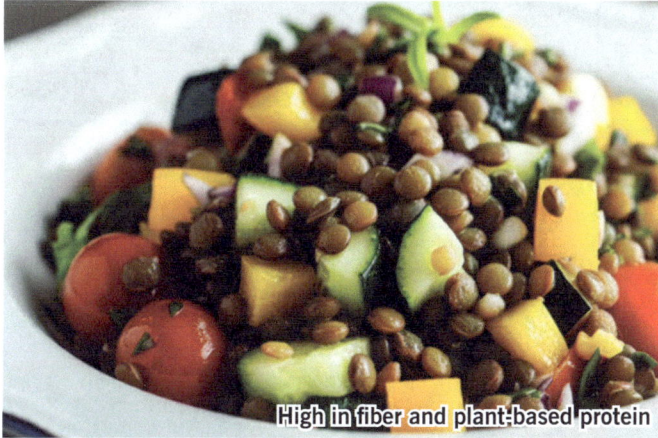

High in fiber and plant-based protein

4 servings

Prep Time **10 min**

Cook Time **20 min**

Nutritional
Calories: 200 kcal
Protein: 10g
Fats: 8g
Carbs: 25g

Instructions

1. In a pot, combine lentils and water. Bring to a boil, then simmer for 20 minutes or until tender. Drain and cool.

2. In a bowl, combine cooked lentils, cherry tomatoes, cucumber, red onion, and parsley.

3. Drizzle with olive oil and lemon juice. Season with salt and black pepper.

4. Toss well and serve chilled.

Ingredients

- 1 cup lentils, rinsed
- 2 cups water
- 1 cup cherry tomatoes, halved
- 1/2 cucumber, diced
- 1/4 cup red onion, finely chopped
- 1/4 cup fresh parsley, chopped
- 3 tbsp olive oil
- 2 tbsp lemon juice
- Salt and black pepper to taste

Ingredient Availability

Available at Walmart, Publix, and Whole Foods.

Chicken Caesar Salad with Greek Yogurt Dressing

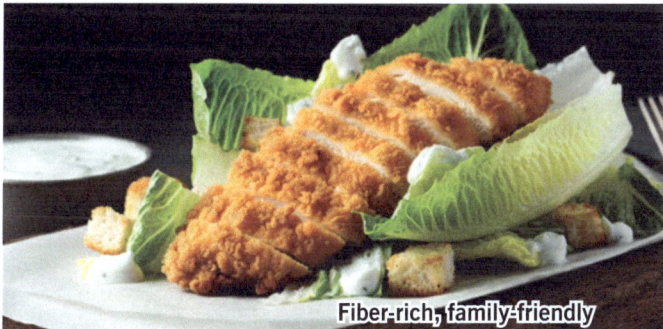

Fiber-rich, family-friendly

4 servings

Prep Time **15 min**

Cook Time **15 min**

Nutritional
Calories: 350 kcal
Protein: 30g
Fats: 15g
Carbs: 20g

Instructions

1. In a bowl, whisk together Greek yogurt, lemon juice, Dijon mustard, garlic, salt, and pepper for the dressing.

2. Toss romaine lettuce with dressing and top with sliced chicken, Parmesan, and croutons.

3. Serve immediately.

Ingredients

- 2 chicken breasts, grilled and sliced
- 4 cups romaine lettuce, chopped
- 1/4 cup grated Parmesan cheese
- 1/2 cup croutons
- 1/2 cup Greek yogurt
- 2 tbsp lemon juice
- 1 tbsp Dijon mustard
- 1 garlic clove, minced
- Salt and black pepper to taste

Ingredient Availability

Found at Target, Harris Teeter, and Aldi.

Grilled Shrimp Salad with Avocado

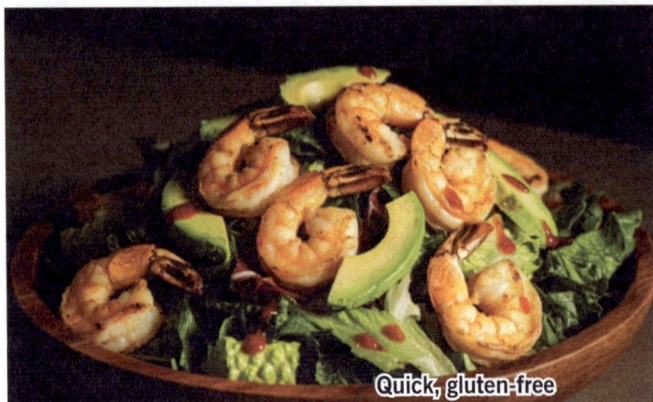

Quick, gluten-free

2 servings

Prep Time **10** min

Cook Time **5** min

Nutritional
Calories: 300 kcal
Protein: 25g
Fats: 20g
Carbs: 12g

Instructions

1. Heat 1 tbsp olive oil in a skillet over medium heat. Cook shrimp for 2-3 minutes on each side until pink.

2. In a large bowl, combine mixed greens, avocado, and cherry tomatoes.

3. Add cooked shrimp, drizzle with remaining olive oil and lemon juice, and season with salt and pepper.

4. Toss gently and serve.

Ingredients

- 1/2 lb shrimp, peeled and deveined
- 1 avocado, diced
- 2 cups mixed greens
- 1/2 cup cherry tomatoes, halved
- 2 tbsp olive oil
- 1 tbsp lemon juice
- Salt and black pepper to taste

Ingredient Availability

Available at Aldi, Whole Foods, and Costco.

Chickpea and Quinoa Salad

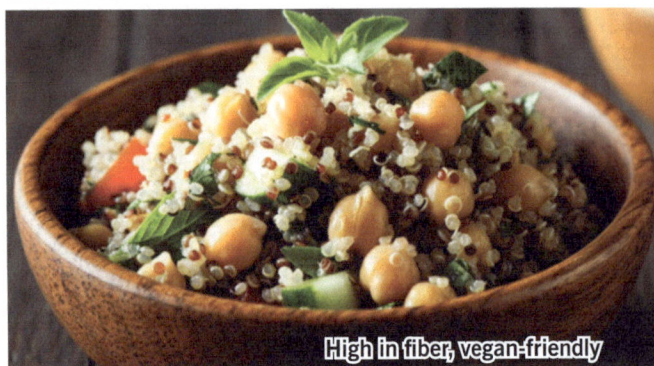

High in fiber, vegan-friendly

4 servings

Prep Time **15** min

Cook Time **15** min

Nutritional
Calories: 250 kcal
Protein: 8g
Fats: 10g
Carbs: 35g

Instructions

1. Combine cooked quinoa, chickpeas, cucumber, bell pepper, and cilantro in a bowl.

2. Drizzle with olive oil and lemon juice. Season with salt and pepper.

3. Toss and serve chilled or at room temperature.

Ingredients

- 1 cup quinoa, cooked
- 1 can chickpeas, drained and rinsed
- 1/2 cucumber, diced
- 1/4 cup red bell pepper, diced
- 1/4 cup fresh cilantro, chopped
- 2 tbsp lemon juice
- 3 tbsp olive oil
- Salt and black pepper to taste

Ingredient Availability

Available at Walmart, Target, and Aldi.

Turkey and Spinach Wraps

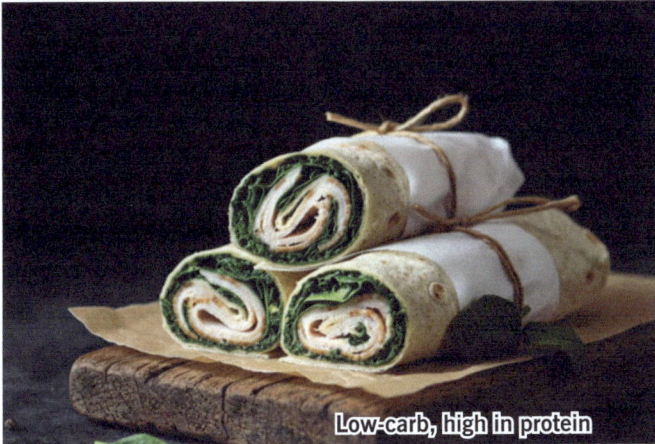

4 wraps

Prep Time **10** min

Cook Time **0** min

Nutritional
Calories: 300 kcal
Protein: 20g
Fats: 12g
Carbs: 30g

Instructions

1. Spread hummus evenly on each wrap.

2. Layer with turkey slices, spinach leaves, and avocado.

3. Season with salt and black pepper, then roll up each wrap tightly.

4. Cut in half and serve.

Low-carb, high in protein

Ingredients

- 4 whole-grain wraps
- 8 slices of turkey breast
- 2 cups spinach leaves
- 1/2 avocado, thinly sliced
- 1/4 cup hummus
- Salt and black pepper to taste

Ingredient Availability

Found at Publix, Whole Foods, and Harris Teeter.

Zucchini Noodles with Pesto

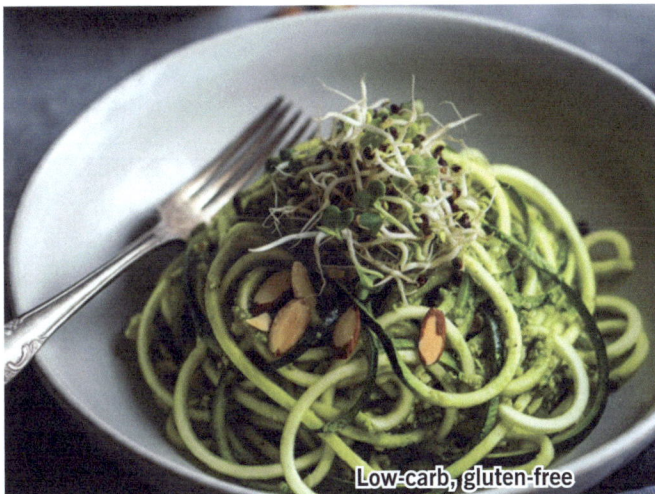

2 servings

Prep Time **10** min

Cook Time **5** min

Nutritional
Calories: 200 kcal
Protein: 6g
Fats: 14g
Carbs: 15g

Instructions

1. Heat a large skillet over medium heat and sauté zucchini noodles for 2 minutes.

2. Add pesto and toss until evenly coated.

3. Top with cherry tomatoes and Parmesan. Season with salt and pepper.

4. Serve immediately.

Low-carb, gluten-free

Ingredients

- 2 medium zucchinis, spiralized
- 1/4 cup basil pesto (store-bought or homemade)
- 1/4 cup cherry tomatoes, halved
- 2 tbsp Parmesan cheese, grated
- Salt and black pepper to taste

Ingredient Availability

Available at Costco, Aldi, and Whole Foods.

Tuna Salad with Lemon and Dill

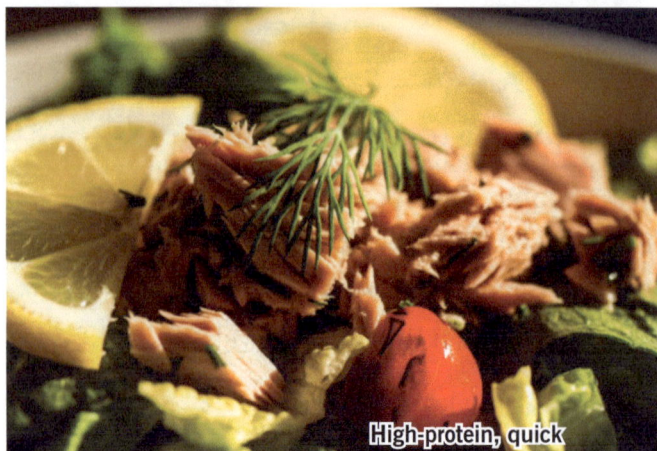
High-protein, quick

2 servings

Prep Time **10** min

Cook Time **0** min

Nutritional
Calories: 180 kcal
Protein: 25g
Fats: 3g
Carbs: 5g

Instructions

1. In a bowl, mix tuna, Greek yogurt, dill, and lemon juice.
2. Season with salt and black pepper.
3. Serve on lettuce leaves or in a sandwich.

Ingredients

- 1 can tuna in water, drained
- 2 tbsp Greek yogurt
- 1 tbsp fresh dill, chopped
- 1 tbsp lemon juice
- Salt and black pepper to taste
- Lettuce leaves for serving

Ingredient Availability

Found at Walmart, Target, and Publix.

Grilled Chicken and Mango Salad

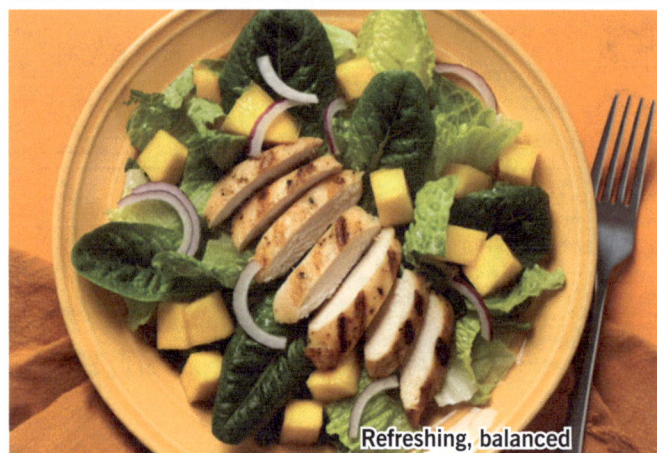
Refreshing, balanced

4 servings

Prep Time **15** min

Cook Time **10** min

Nutritional
Calories: 320 kcal
Protein: 25g
Fats: 10g
Carbs: 28g

Instructions

1. In a large bowl, combine mixed greens, mango, and red onion.
2. Top with grilled chicken and drizzle with balsamic vinaigrette.
3. Season with salt and black pepper and serve.

Ingredients

- 2 chicken breasts, grilled and sliced
- 2 cups mixed greens
- 1 mango, diced
- 1/4 cup red onion, thinly sliced
- 3 tbsp balsamic vinaigrette
- Salt and black pepper to taste

Ingredient Availability

Available at Publix, Whole Foods, and Costco.

Kale Salad with Cranberries and Almonds

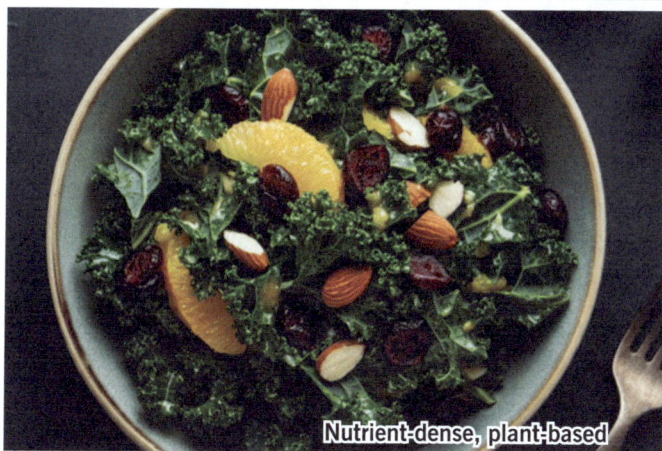

Nutrient-dense, plant-based

4 servings

Prep Time **10** min

Cook Time **0** min

Nutritional
Calories: 180 kcal
Protein: 5g
Fats: 12g
Carbs: 15g

Instructions

1. In a large bowl, massage kale with lemon juice and olive oil for 2-3 minutes until tender.

2. Add cranberries and almonds, and toss.

3. Season with salt and black pepper, then serve.

Ingredients

- 4 cups kale, chopped
- 1/4 cup dried cranberries
- 1/4 cup sliced almonds
- 2 tbsp lemon juice
- 2 tbsp olive oil
- Salt and black pepper to taste

Ingredient Availability

Available at Aldi, Target, and Walmart.

Mediterranean Couscous Bowl

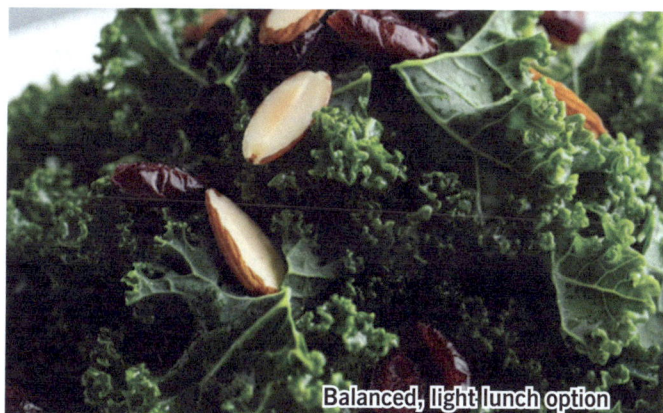

Balanced, light lunch option

4 servings

Prep Time **15** min

Cook Time **10** min

Nutritional
Calories: 250 kcal
Protein: 8g
Fats: 10g
Carbs: 32g

Instructions

1. In a large bowl, combine couscous, cherry tomatoes, cucumber, feta cheese, olives, and red onion.

2. Drizzle with lemon juice and olive oil, then toss well.

3. Season with salt and black pepper, then serve.

Ingredients

- 1 cup cooked couscous
- 1/2 cup cherry tomatoes, halved
- 1/2 cucumber, diced
- 1/4 cup feta cheese, crumbled
- 1/4 cup black olives, sliced
- 2 tbsp red onion, finely chopped
- 2 tbsp lemon juice
- 2 tbsp olive oil
- Salt and black pepper to taste

Ingredient Availability

Available at Publix, Costco, and Whole Foods.

Cucumber and Hummus Sandwich

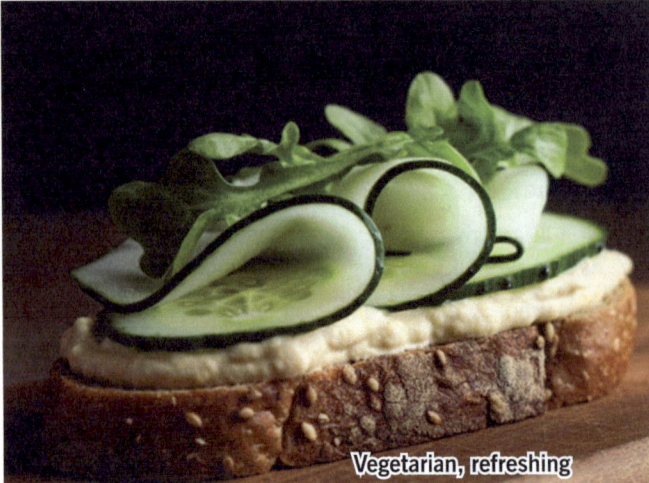

Vegetarian, refreshing

2 servings		**Nutritional**
Prep Time **10** min		Calories: 250 kcal Protein: 9g
Cook Time **0** min		Fats: 8g Carbs: 35g

Instructions

1. Spread hummus on each slice of bread.
2. Layer cucumber slices and alfalfa sprouts on two slices, season with salt and black pepper.
3. Top with the remaining slices of bread and serve.

Ingredients

- 4 slices whole-grain bread
- 1/2 cup hummus
- 1/2 cucumber, thinly sliced
- 1/4 cup alfalfa sprouts
- Salt and black pepper to taste

Ingredient Availability

Found at Whole Foods, Harris Teeter, and Walmart.

Vegetable Wrap with Hummus

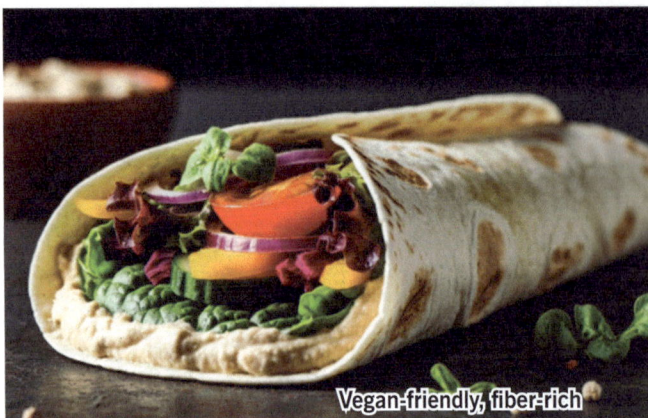

Vegan-friendly, fiber-rich

4 wraps		**Nutritional**
Prep Time **15** min		Calories: 300 kcal Protein: 10g
Cook Time **0** min		Fats: 10g Carbs: 40g

Instructions

1. Spread hummus on each wrap.
2. Layer bell pepper, carrots, cucumber, and spinach.
3. Season with salt and black pepper, then roll up tightly.
4. Cut in half and serve.

Ingredients

- 4 whole-grain wraps
- 1 cup hummus
- 1/2 cup red bell pepper, thinly sliced
- 1/2 cup shredded carrots
- 1/2 cup cucumber, thinly sliced
- 1/4 cup spinach leaves
- Salt and black pepper to taste

Ingredient Availability

Available at Aldi, Costco, and Publix.

Spicy Black Bean and Corn Salad

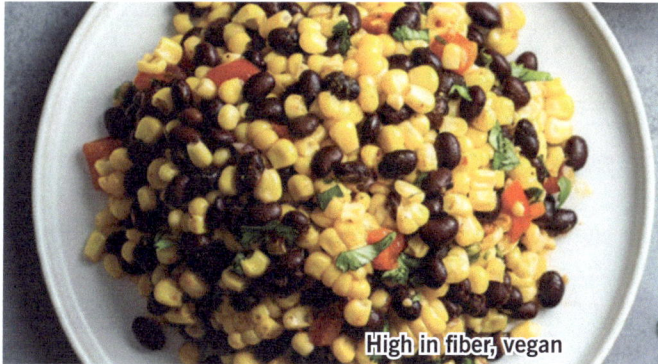

4 servings

Prep Time **15** min

Cook Time **0** min

Nutritional
Calories: 220 kcal
Protein: 8g
Fats: 6g
Carbs: 35g

High in fiber, vegan

Instructions

1. In a bowl, combine black beans, corn, cherry tomatoes, red onion, and cilantro.
2. Drizzle with lime juice and olive oil, then add cumin, salt, and black pepper.
3. Toss well and serve chilled or at room temperature.

Ingredients

- 1 cup corn kernels (fresh or canned)
- 1/2 cup cherry tomatoes, halved
- 1/4 cup red onion, diced
- 2 tbsp cilantro, chopped
- 2 tbsp lime juice
- 1 tbsp olive oil
- 1/2 tsp cumin
- Salt and black pepper to taste

Ingredient Availability

Available at Walmart, Aldi, and Harris Teeter.

Tabbouleh with Grilled Chicken

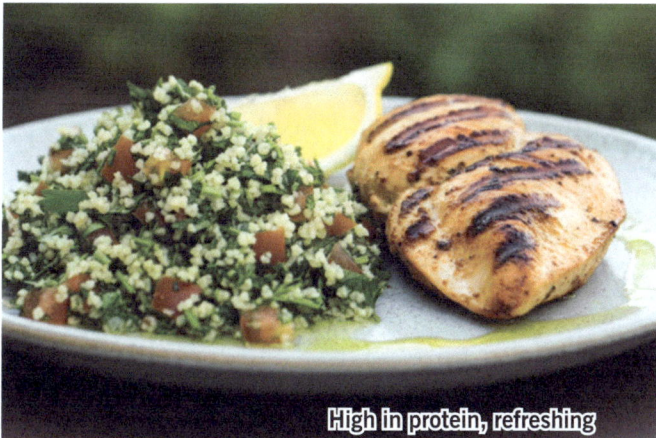

4 servings

Prep Time **15** min

Cook Time **15** min

Nutritional
Calories: 350 kcal
Protein: 30g
Fats: 12g
Carbs: 35g

High in protein, refreshing

Instructions

1. In a large bowl, mix cooked bulgur, parsley, mint, tomatoes, and cucumber.
2. Drizzle with lemon juice and olive oil, season with salt and black pepper, and toss.
3. Top with sliced grilled chicken and serve.

Ingredients

- 1 cup cooked bulgur
- 2 grilled chicken breasts, sliced
- 1/2 cup parsley, chopped
- 1/4 cup mint leaves, chopped
- 2 tomatoes, diced
- 1/2 cucumber, diced
- 3 tbsp lemon juice
- 3 tbsp olive oil
- Salt and black pepper to taste

Ingredient Availability

Found at Target, Costco, and Whole Foods.

Tomato Basil Soup with Grilled Cheese

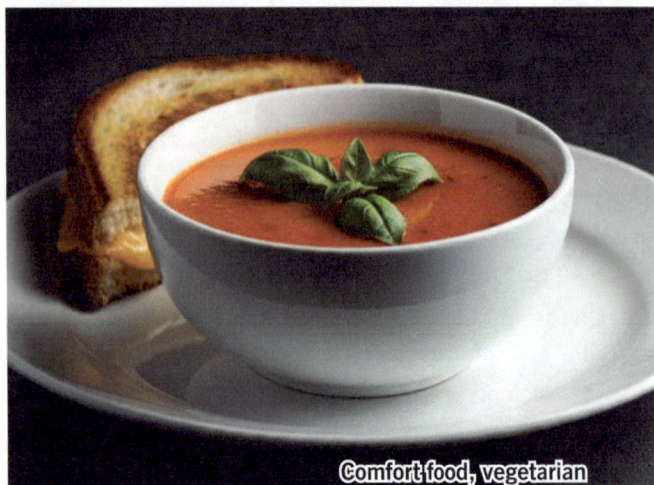

Comfort food, vegetarian

4 servings

Prep Time **10** min

Cook Time **20** min

Nutritional
Calories: 400 kcal
Protein: 15g
Fats: 18g
Carbs: 45g

Instructions

1. Heat tomato soup according to package instructions.
2. Butter one side of each slice of bread. Place cheese and basil between two slices and grill until golden brown.
3. Serve the soup with grilled cheese on the side.

Ingredients

- 4 cups tomato soup (homemade or store-bought)
- 8 slices whole-grain bread
- 4 slices cheddar cheese
- 1/4 cup fresh basil leaves
- 2 tbsp butter

Ingredient Availability

Available at Publix, Walmart, and Aldi.

Grilled Salmon Salad with Spinach

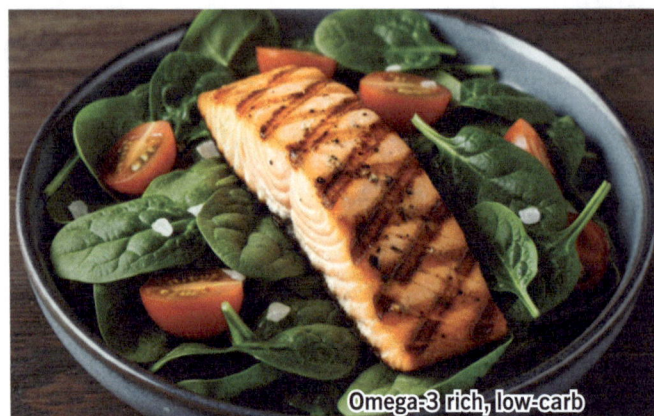

Omega-3 rich, low-carb

2 servings

Prep Time **15** min

Cook Time **10** min

Nutritional
Calories: 450 kcal
Protein: 35g
Fats: 30g
Carbs: 10g

Instructions

1. Grill salmon fillets for 4-5 minutes on each side.
2. Arrange spinach, avocado, and cherry tomatoes in a bowl.
3. Place salmon on top, drizzle with lemon juice and olive oil, and season with salt and black pepper.
4. Serve immediately.

Ingredients

- 2 salmon fillets
- 4 cups baby spinach
- 1/2 avocado, sliced
- 1/4 cup cherry tomatoes, halved
- 2 tbsp lemon juice
- 2 tbsp olive oil
- Salt and black pepper to taste

Ingredient Availability

Found at Whole Foods, Harris Teeter, and Costco.

Quinoa and Beet Salad

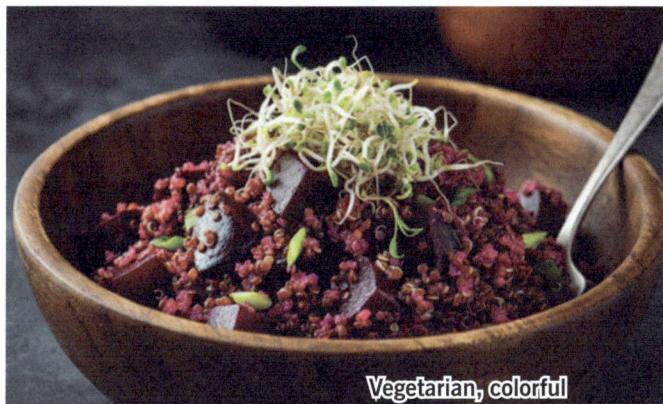

4 servings

Prep Time **15 min**

Cook Time **10 min**

Nutritional
Calories: 320 kcal
Protein: 10g
Fats: 14g
Carbs: 35g

Vegetarian, colorful

Instructions

1. In a large bowl, mix quinoa, beets, goat cheese, and walnuts.
2. Drizzle with balsamic vinegar and olive oil, then season with salt and black pepper.
3. Toss gently and serve.

Ingredients

- 1 cup cooked quinoa
- 1/2 cup cooked beets, diced
- 1/4 cup goat cheese, crumbled
- 2 tbsp walnuts, chopped
- 2 tbsp balsamic vinegar
- 2 tbsp olive oil
- Salt and black pepper to taste

Ingredient Availability

Available at Aldi, Publix, and Whole Foods.

Caprese Salad with Balsamic Glaze

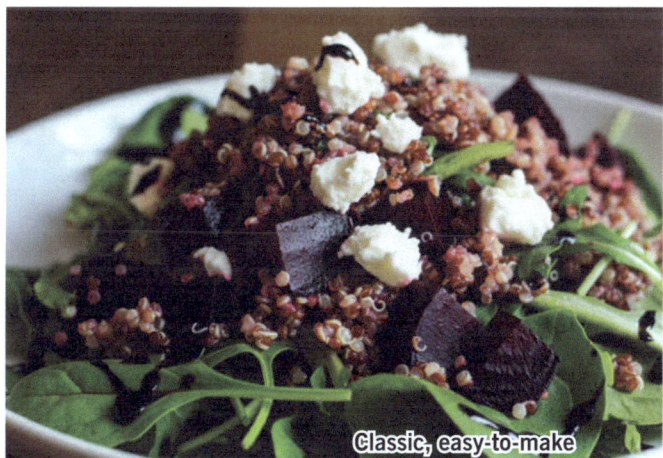

2 servings

Prep Time **10 min**

Cook Time **0 min**

Nutritional
Calories: 250 kcal
Protein: 12g
Fats: 18g
Carbs: 10g

Classic, easy-to-make

Instructions

1. Alternate layers of tomato and mozzarella slices on a serving plate.
2. Add basil leaves between the slices.
3. Drizzle with balsamic glaze and olive oil, and season with salt and black pepper.
4. Serve immediately.

Ingredients

- 2 large tomatoes, sliced
- 8 oz fresh mozzarella, sliced
- 1/4 cup fresh basil leaves
- 2 tbsp balsamic glaze
- 1 tbsp olive oil
- Salt and black pepper to taste

Ingredient Availability

Found at Costco, Walmart, and Whole Foods.

Soba Noodle Salad with Sesame Dressing

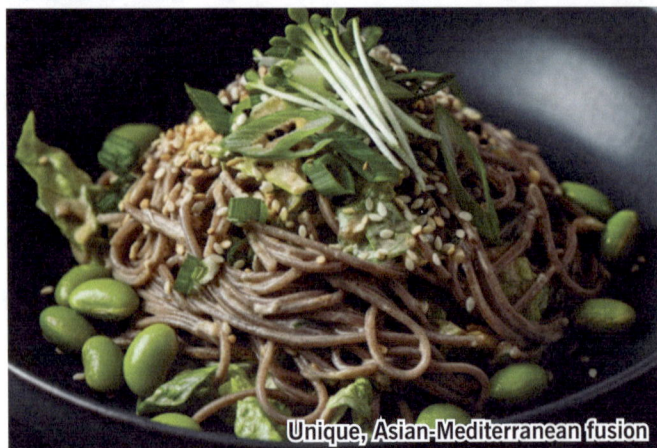

4 servings

Prep Time **15** min

Cook Time **5** min

Nutritional
Calories: 280 kcal
Protein: 10g
Fats: 10g
Carbs: 40g

Unique, Asian-Mediterranean fusion

Instructions

1. In a bowl, whisk sesame oil, soy sauce, rice vinegar, and honey for the dressing.
2. Combine soba noodles, red cabbage, cucumber, and edamame in a serving bowl.
3. Pour dressing over the salad, toss to combine, and garnish with sesame seeds.
4. Serve chilled.

Ingredients

- 8 oz soba noodles, cooked and cooled
- 1/2 cup red cabbage, shredded
- 1/2 cucumber, julienned
- 1/4 cup edamame

- 2 tbsp sesame oil
- 1 tbsp soy sauce
- 1 tbsp rice vinegar
- 1 tsp honey
- Sesame seeds for garnish

Ingredient Availability

Found at Whole Foods, Publix, and Walmart.

Chickpea Curry with Spinach

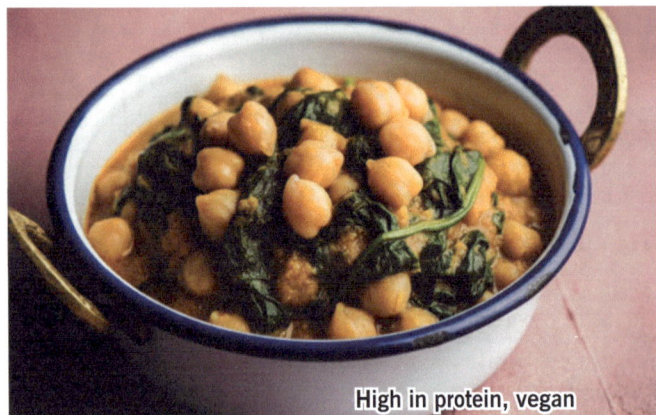

4 servings

Prep Time **10** min

Cook Time **20** min

Nutritional
Calories: 220 kcal
Protein: 8g
Fats: 12g
Carbs: 20g

High in protein, vegan

Instructions

1. Heat olive oil in a pot over medium heat. Add curry powder and sauté for 1 minute.
2. Stir in chickpeas, tomatoes, and coconut milk. Simmer for 10 minutes.
3. Add spinach, cook until wilted. Season with salt and black pepper.
4. Serve over rice or as is.

Ingredients

- 1 can chickpeas, drained and rinsed
- 2 cups fresh spinach
- 1/2 cup coconut milk
- 1/4 cup diced tomatoes
- 2 tbsp curry powder
- 1 tbsp olive oil
- Salt and black pepper to taste

Ingredient Availability

Available at Aldi, Costco, and Publix.

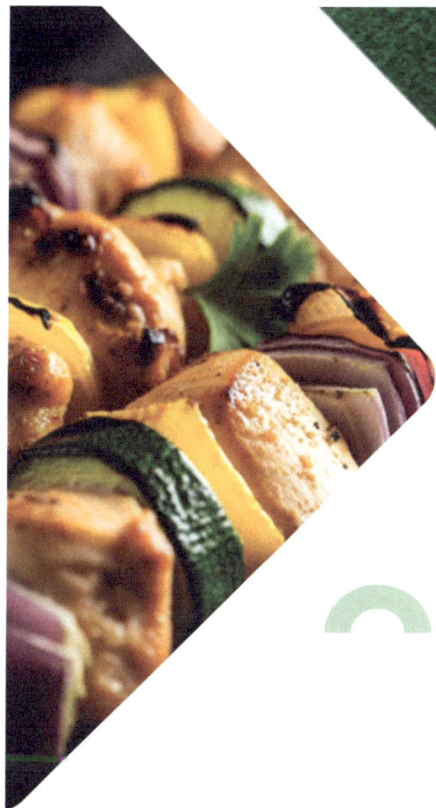

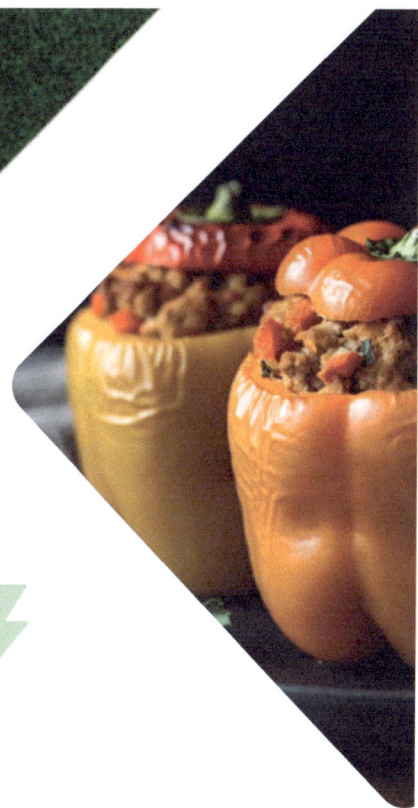

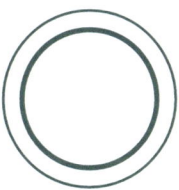

Chapter 5
Dinner Recipes

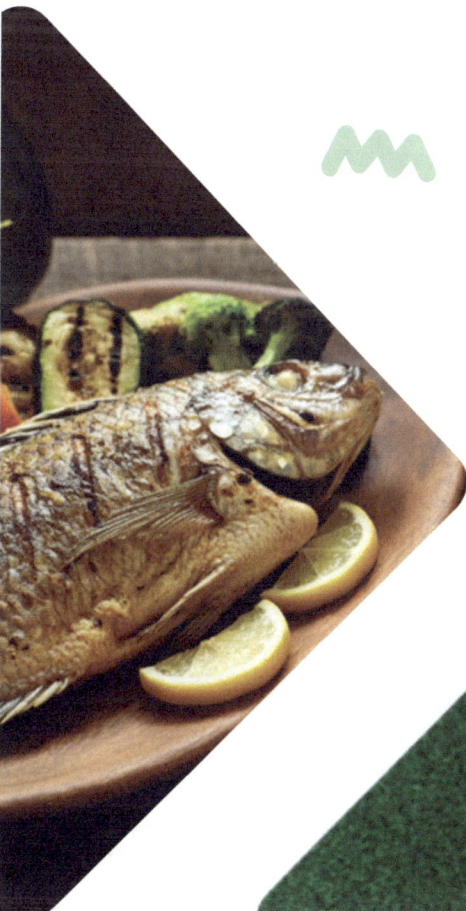

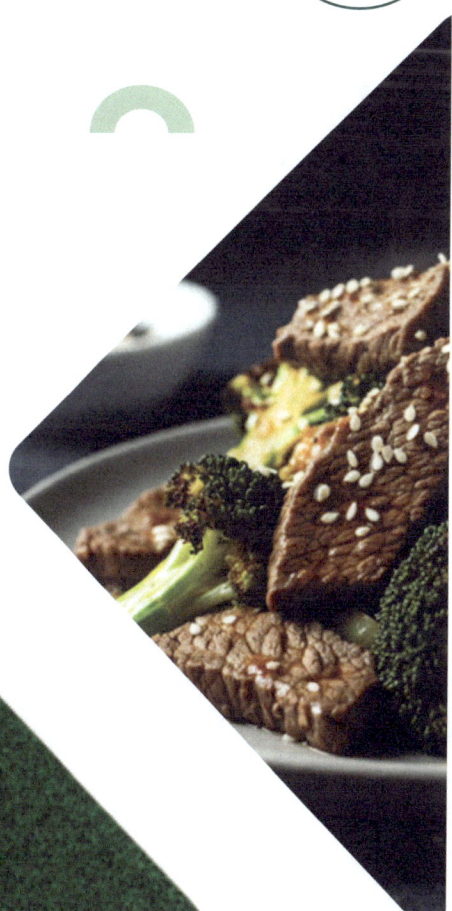

Lemon Herb Chicken with Brown Rice

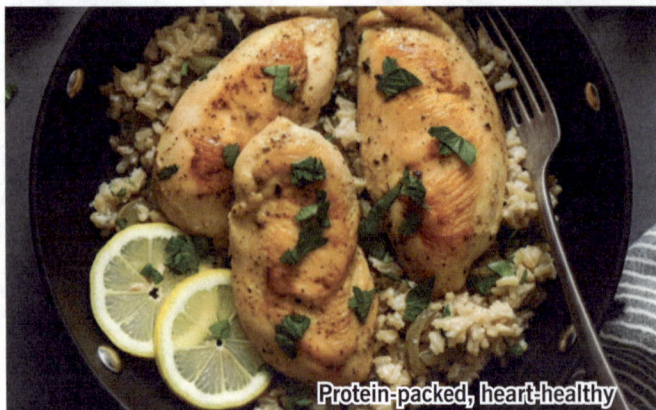
Protein-packed, heart-healthy

4 servings

Prep Time **15** min

Cook Time **30** min

Nutritional
Calories: 350 kcal
Protein: 35g
Fats: 10g
Carbs: 40g

Instructions

1. In a bowl, whisk sesame oil, soy sauce, rice vinegar, and honey for the dressing.

2. Combine soba noodles, red cabbage, cucumber, and edamame in a serving bowl.

3. Pour dressing over the salad, toss to combine, and garnish with sesame seeds.

4. Serve chilled.

Ingredients

- 4 boneless, skinless chicken breasts
- 2 tbsp lemon juice
- 1 tbsp olive oil
- 2 tsp dried oregano
- 1 cup brown rice, cooked
- 1 cup steamed broccoli
- Salt and pepper to taste

Ingredient Availability

Found at Aldi, Target, and Walmart.

Grilled Tilapia with Garlic and Lemon

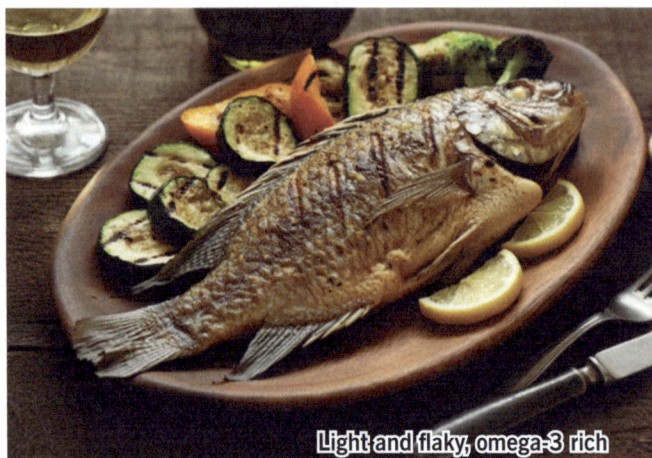
Light and flaky, omega-3 rich

4 servings

Prep Time **10** min

Cook Time **10** min

Nutritional
Calories: 220 kcal
Protein: 25g
Fats: 10g
Carbs: 2g

Instructions

1. Preheat grill to medium-high heat. Season tilapia with garlic, lemon juice, olive oil, salt, and pepper.

2. Grill fillets for 4-5 minutes per side or until cooked through.

3. Serve with lemon wedges.

Ingredients

- 4 tilapia fillets
- 2 cloves garlic, minced
- 2 tbsp lemon juice
- 1 tbsp olive oil
- Salt and black pepper to taste
- Lemon wedges for serving

Ingredient Availability

Available at Whole Foods, Publix, and Walmart.

Baked Cod with Cherry Tomatoes

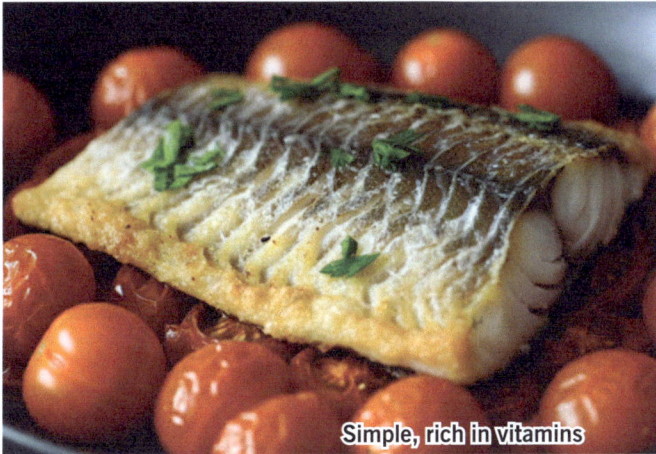
Simple, rich in vitamins

4 servings

Prep Time **10** min

Cook Time **20** min

Nutritional
Calories: 250 kcal
Protein: 30g
Fats: 12g
Carbs: 5g

Instructions

1. Preheat oven to 400°F (200°C). Place cod fillets and cherry tomatoes in a baking dish.
2. Drizzle with olive oil, sprinkle with garlic, salt, and pepper.
3. Bake for 15-20 minutes or until fish is opaque and flakes easily.
4. Garnish with fresh basil before serving.

Ingredients

- 4 cod fillets
- 1 cup cherry tomatoes, halved
- 2 tbsp olive oil
- 1 clove garlic, minced
- Salt and pepper to taste
- Fresh basil for garnish

Ingredient Availability

Available at Costco, Aldi, and Whole Foods.

Beef Stir-Fry with Broccoli

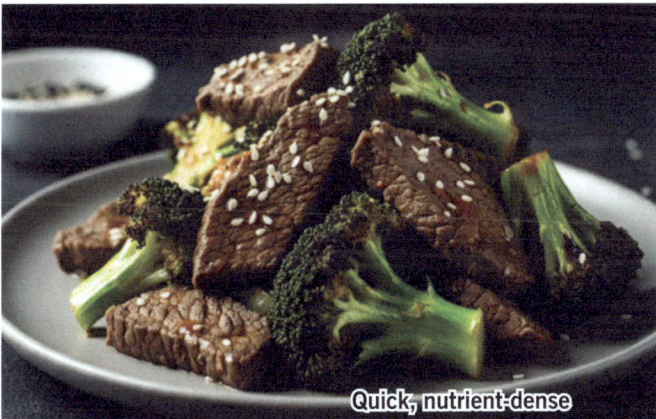
Quick, nutrient-dense

4 servings

Prep Time **15** min

Cook Time **10** min

Nutritional
Calories: 350 kcal
Protein: 28g
Fats: 18g
Carbs: 15g

Instructions

1. Heat olive oil in a large skillet over medium-high heat. Add beef strips and cook for 3-4 minutes.
2. Add broccoli, bell pepper, soy sauce, and ginger. Stir-fry for 5-6 minutes or until vegetables are tender-crisp.
3. Season with salt and black pepper, and serve.

Ingredients

- 1 lb lean beef strips
- 2 cups broccoli florets
- 1 red bell pepper, sliced
- 2 tbsp soy sauce (low sodium)
- 1 tbsp olive oil
- 1 tsp ginger, minced
- Salt and black pepper to taste

Ingredient Availability

Found at Walmart, Aldi, and Publix.

Chicken and Vegetable Skewers

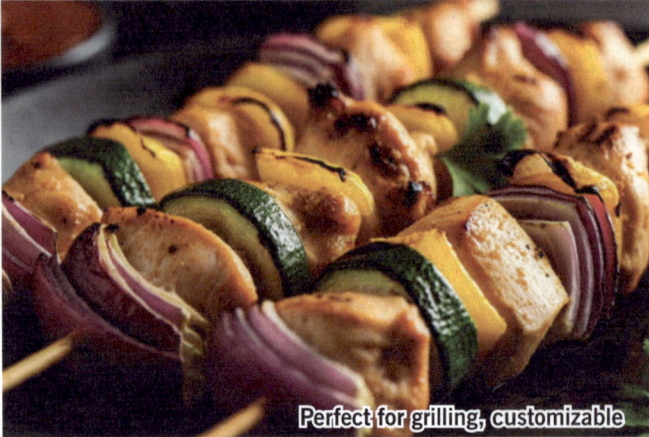

Perfect for grilling, customizable

4 servings

Prep Time **20** min

Cook Time **15** min

Nutritional
Calories: 300 kcal
Protein: 25g
Fats: 14g
Carbs: 12g

Instructions

1. Preheat grill to medium heat. Thread chicken, bell pepper, zucchini, and onion onto skewers.

2. Brush with olive oil, lemon juice, and paprika. Season with salt and black pepper.

3. Grill for 10-15 minutes, turning occasionally, until chicken is cooked through.

4. Serve with a side salad or rice.

Ingredients

- 2 chicken breasts, cubed
- 1 red bell pepper, cut into chunks
- 1 zucchini, sliced
- 1 red onion, cut into wedges
- 2 tbsp olive oil
- 1 tbsp lemon juice
- 1 tsp paprika
- Salt and black pepper to taste

Ingredient Availability

Found at Aldi, Costco, and Target.

Herb-Crusted Pork Tenderloin

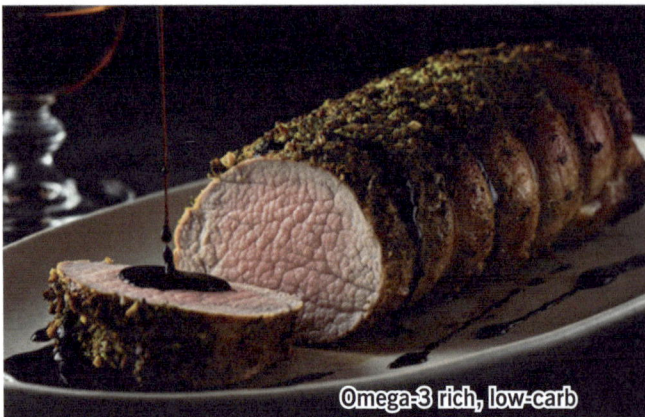

Omega-3 rich, low-carb

4 servings

Prep Time **15** min

Cook Time **25** min

Nutritional
Calories: 350 kcal
Protein: 28g
Fats: 14g
Carbs: 20g

Instructions

1. Preheat oven to 425°F (220°C). Coat pork tenderloin with Dijon mustard.

2. In a bowl, mix breadcrumbs, rosemary, thyme, salt, and pepper.

3. Roll the pork in the breadcrumb mixture until coated.

4. Place on a baking sheet and roast for 25 minutes or until internal temperature reaches 145°F (63°C).

5. Let rest for 5 minutes before slicing and serving.

Ingredients

- 1 pork tenderloin
- 2 tbsp Dijon mustard
- 1 tbsp olive oil
- 1/2 cup breadcrumbs
- 1 tbsp fresh rosemary, chopped
- 1 tbsp fresh thyme, chopped
- Salt and black pepper to taste

Ingredient Availability

Available at Publix, Whole Foods, and Walmart.

Stuffed Bell Peppers with Ground Turkey

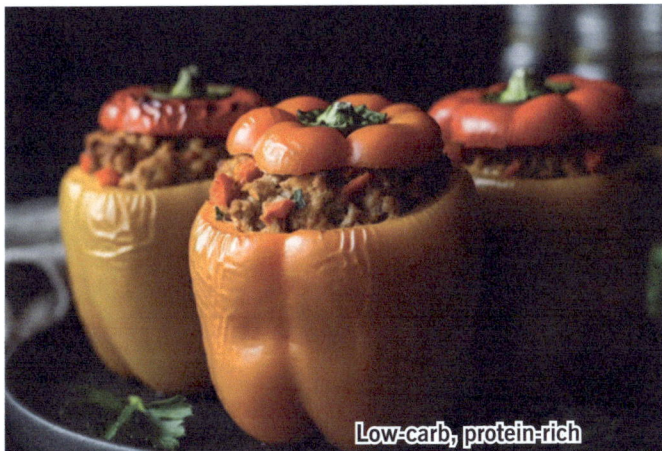

Low-carb, protein-rich

4 servings

Prep Time **15 min**

Cook Time **30 min**

Nutritional
Calories: 300 kcal
Protein: 28g
Fats: 10g
Carbs: 25g

Instructions

1. Preheat oven to 375°F (190°C). In a skillet, cook ground turkey until browned. Mix with cooked rice, tomato sauce, garlic powder, salt, and pepper.

2. Stuff each bell pepper with the turkey mixture and place in a baking dish.

3. Sprinkle mozzarella on top and bake for 25-30 minutes or until peppers are tender.

4. Serve with a side salad or steamed vegetables.

Ingredients

- 4 large bell peppers, tops cut off and seeds removed
- 1 lb ground turkey
- 1/2 cup cooked brown rice
- 1/2 cup tomato sauce
- 1/4 cup shredded mozzarella
- 1 tsp garlic powder
- Salt and black pepper to taste

Ingredient Availability

Found at Target, Aldi, and Whole Foods.

Baked Eggplant Parmesan

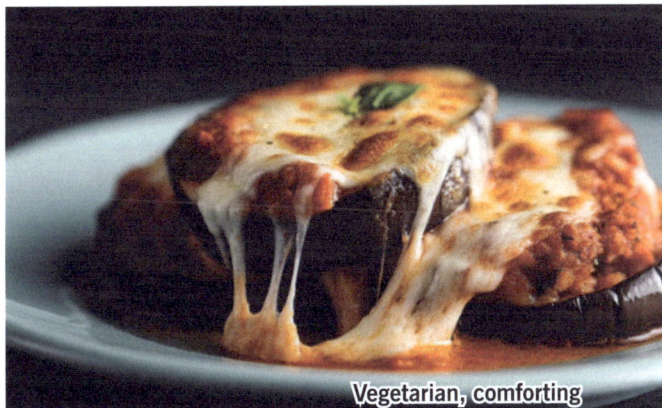

Vegetarian, comforting

4 servings

Prep Time **20 min**

Cook Time **30 min**

Nutritional
Calories: 320 kcal
Protein: 14g
Fats: 16g
Carbs: 30g

Instructions

1. Preheat oven to 400°F (200°C). Brush eggplant slices with olive oil, season with salt and pepper.

2. Dip each slice in the beaten egg, then coat with a mixture of breadcrumbs and Parmesan cheese.

3. Place on a baking sheet and bake for 20 minutes, flipping halfway through.

4. Top each slice with marinara sauce and mozzarella cheese, then bake for another 10 minutes until cheese is melted.

5. Garnish with fresh basil and serve

Ingredients

- 2 large eggplants, sliced into rounds
- 1 cup breadcrumbs
- 1/2 cup grated Parmesan cheese
- 1 cup marinara sauce
- 1 cup shredded mozzarella cheese
- 1 egg, beaten
- 2 tbsp olive oil
- Salt and black pepper to taste
- Fresh basil leaves for garnish

Ingredient Availability

Found at Aldi, Publix, and Whole Foods.

Vegetable Stir-Fry with Tofu

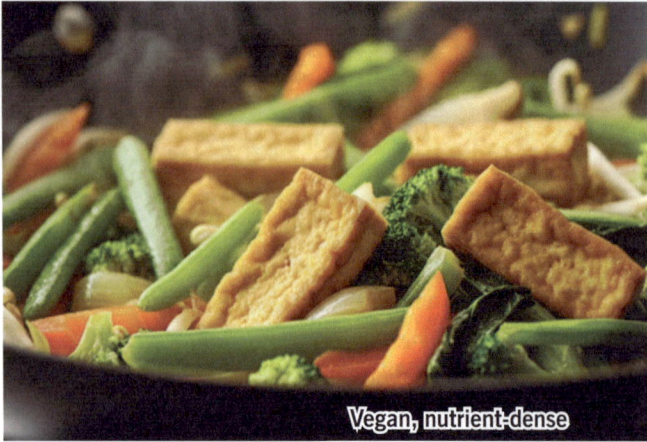

Vegan, nutrient-dense

		Nutritional
4 servings		Calories: 250 kcal
Prep Time **15** min		Protein: 12g
		Fats: 14g
Cook Time **15** min		Carbs: 18g

Instructions

1. Heat sesame oil in a large skillet over medium-high heat. Add tofu and cook until golden brown.

2. Add garlic and ginger, stir for 1 minute.

3. Add mixed vegetables and soy sauce. Stir-fry for 5-7 minutes until vegetables are tender-crisp.

4. Season with salt and pepper. Garnish with sesame seeds before serving.

Ingredients

- 1 block firm tofu, cubed
- 2 cups mixed vegetables (broccoli, carrots, bell peppers)
- 2 tbsp soy sauce (low sodium)
- 1 tbsp sesame oil
- 1 clove garlic, minced
- 1 tsp grated ginger
- Salt and black pepper to taste
- Sesame seeds for garnish

Ingredient Availability

Available at Walmart, Aldi, and Whole Foods.

Roasted Lamb with Rosemary and Thyme

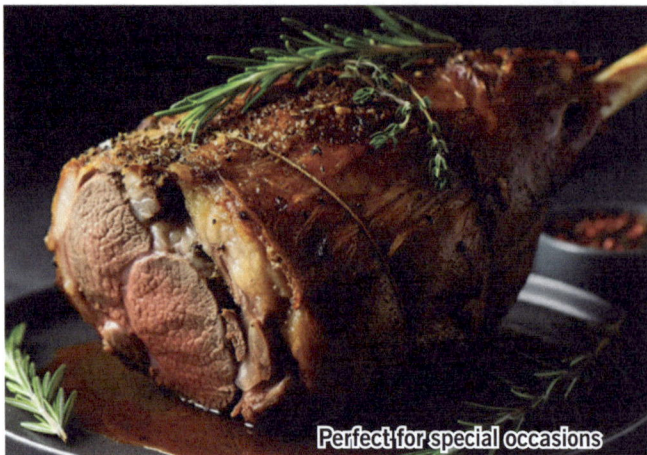

Perfect for special occasions

		Nutritional
4 servings		Calories: 450 kcal
Prep Time **15** min		Protein: 35g
		Fats: 30g
Cook Time **1** h		Carbs: 2g

Instructions

1. Preheat oven to 375°F (190°C). Rub the lamb with olive oil, garlic, rosemary, thyme, salt, and pepper.

2. Place in a roasting pan and bake for 1 hour or until the internal temperature reaches 145°F (63°C).

3. Let rest for 10 minutes before slicing and serving.

Ingredients

- 2 lb lamb leg or shoulder
- 2 tbsp olive oil
- 2 cloves garlic, minced
- 1 tbsp fresh rosemary, chopped
- 1 tbsp fresh thyme, chopped
- Salt and black pepper to taste

Ingredient Availability

Found at Costco, Publix, and Target.

Mediterranean Chicken with Olives

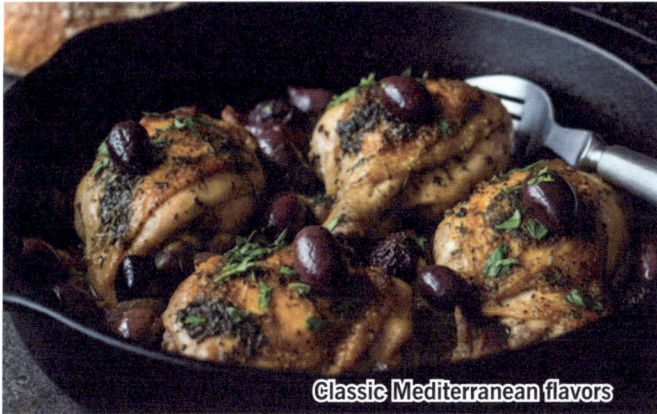

Classic Mediterranean flavors

4 servings

Prep Time **10** min

Cook Time **30** min

Nutritional
Calories: 380 kcal
Protein: 28g
Fats: 24g
Carbs: 4g

Ingredients

- 4 chicken thighs, bone-in, skin-on
- 1/2 cup green olives, pitted and sliced
- 1 lemon, sliced
- 2 tbsp olive oil
- 2 cloves garlic, minced
- 1 tsp dried oregano
- Salt and black pepper to taste

Instructions

1. Preheat oven to 400°F (200°C). Season chicken with salt, pepper, and oregano.

2. Heat olive oil in a skillet over medium-high heat. Sear chicken thighs for 3 minutes per side.

3. Add garlic, lemon slices, and olives. Transfer the skillet to the oven and bake for 20 minutes until chicken is fully cooked.

4. Serve with a side of rice or couscous.

Ingredient Availability

Found at Target, Whole Foods, and Aldi.

Spaghetti Squash with Turkey Marinara

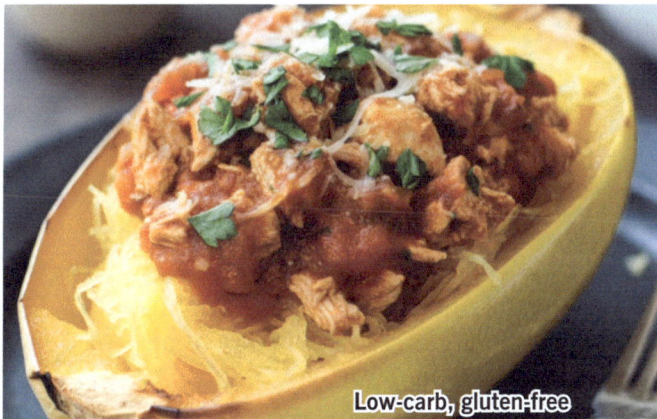

Low-carb, gluten-free

4 servings

Prep Time **15** min

Cook Time **40** min

Nutritional
Calories: 320 kcal
Protein: 28g
Fats: 14g
Carbs: 20g

Ingredients

- 1 large spaghetti squash
- 1 lb ground turkey
- 1 cup marinara sauce (low sodium)
- 2 tbsp olive oil
- 1 clove garlic, minced
- 1/4 cup grated Parmesan cheese
- Salt and black pepper to taste

Instructions

1. Preheat oven to 400°F (200°C). Cut the spaghetti squash in half, remove seeds, and drizzle with olive oil. Bake for 30 minutes, flesh side down.

2. In a skillet, cook ground turkey with garlic until browned. Add marinara sauce, salt, and pepper, and simmer for 10 minutes.

3. Scrape spaghetti squash with a fork to create strands. Top with turkey marinara and Parmesan cheese.

4. Serve warm.

Ingredient Availability

Available at Walmart, Publix, and Costco.

Lemon Garlic Shrimp with Couscous

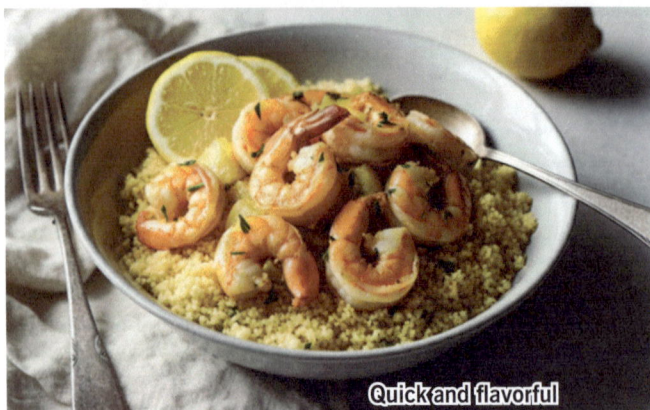

Quick and flavorful

4 servings

Prep Time **10** min

Cook Time **15** min

Nutritional
Calories: 360 kcal
Protein: 25g
Fats: 14g
Carbs: 30g

Instructions

1. Cook couscous according to package instructions. Set aside.

2. Heat olive oil in a skillet over medium heat. Add garlic and shrimp, cooking for 3-4 minutes until pink.

3. Stir in lemon juice, salt, and pepper. Serve shrimp over couscous and garnish with parsley.

Ingredients

- 1 lb large shrimp, peeled and deveined
- 1 cup couscous
- 2 tbsp lemon juice
- 2 tbsp olive oil
- 2 cloves garlic, minced
- Salt and black pepper to taste
- Fresh parsley for garnish

Ingredient Availability

Found at Aldi, Target, and Whole Foods.

Honey Mustard Salmon

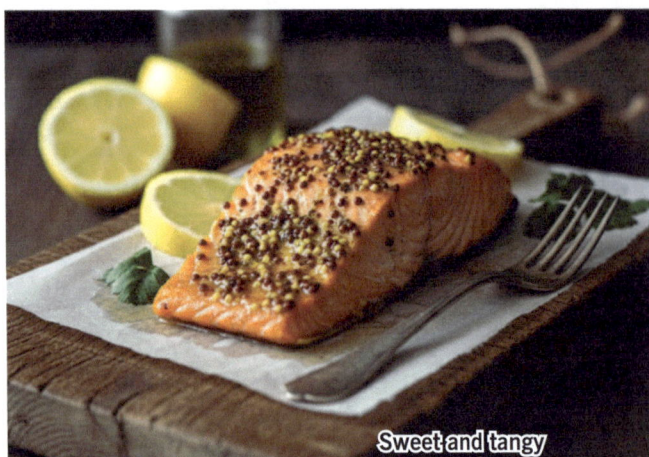

Sweet and tangy

4 servings

Prep Time **5** min

Cook Time **15** min

Nutritional
Calories: 350 kcal
Protein: 30g
Fats: 18g
Carbs: 10g

Instructions

1. Preheat oven to 400°F (200°C). In a small bowl, mix honey, Dijon mustard, and olive oil.

2. Brush salmon fillets with the mixture and place on a baking sheet. Season with salt and pepper.

3. Bake for 12-15 minutes or until salmon is cooked through.

4. Serve with lemon wedges.

Ingredients

- 4 salmon fillets
- 2 tbsp honey
- 1 tbsp Dijon mustard
- 1 tbsp olive oil
- Salt and black pepper to taste
- Lemon wedges for serving

Ingredient Availability

Available at Costco, Walmart, and Whole Foods.

Quinoa Stuffed Portobello Mushrooms

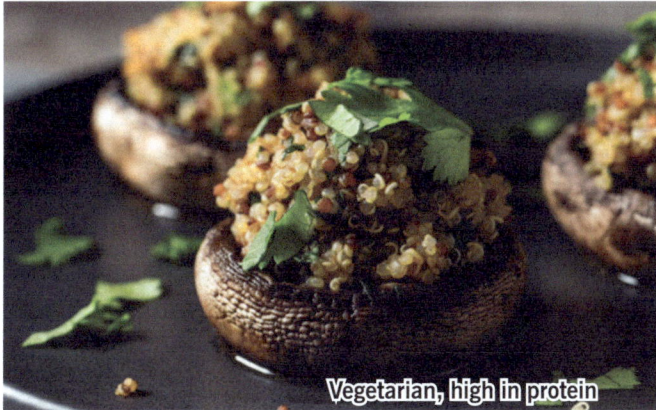

4 servings

Prep Time **15** min

Cook Time **25** min

Nutritional
Calories: 250 kcal
Protein: 10g
Fats: 12g
Carbs: 28g

Vegetarian, high in protein

Ingredients

- 4 large Portobello mushrooms, stems removed
- 1 cup cooked quinoa
- 1/2 cup cherry tomatoes, diced
- 1/4 cup feta cheese, crumbled
- 2 tbsp olive oil
- 1 clove garlic, minced
- 1 tsp dried oregano
- Salt and black pepper to taste
- Fresh parsley for garnish

Instructions

1. Preheat oven to 375°F (190°C). Brush mushrooms with olive oil and place on a baking sheet.
2. In a bowl, mix cooked quinoa, cherry tomatoes, feta cheese, garlic, oregano, salt, and pepper.
3. Stuff each mushroom with the quinoa mixture and bake for 20-25 minutes until mushrooms are tender.
4. Garnish with fresh parsley before serving.

Ingredient Availability

Found at Whole Foods, Aldi, and Publix.

Ratatouille with Fresh Basil

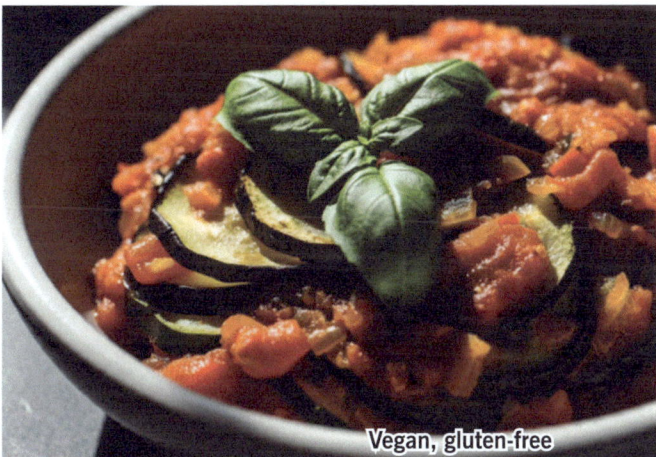

4 servings

Prep Time **15** min

Cook Time **45** min

Nutritional
Calories: 180 kcal
Protein: 3g
Fats: 10g
Carbs: 20g

Vegan, gluten-free

Ingredients

- 1 eggplant, diced
- 1 zucchini, sliced
- 1 bell pepper, chopped
- 1 onion, diced
- 2 cups diced tomatoes (canned or fresh)
- 2 tbsp olive oil
- 2 cloves garlic, minced
- Salt and black pepper to taste
- Fresh basil leaves for garnish

Instructions

1. Preheat oven to 400°F (200°C). In a large baking dish, layer the eggplant, zucchini, bell pepper, and onion.
2. Pour the diced tomatoes over the vegetables and drizzle with olive oil.
3. Sprinkle garlic, salt, and pepper. Cover with foil and bake for 35 minutes.
4. Remove the foil and bake for an additional 10 minutes. Garnish with fresh basil and serve.

Ingredient Availability

Available at Aldi, Target, and Whole Foods.

Chicken Piccata with Capers

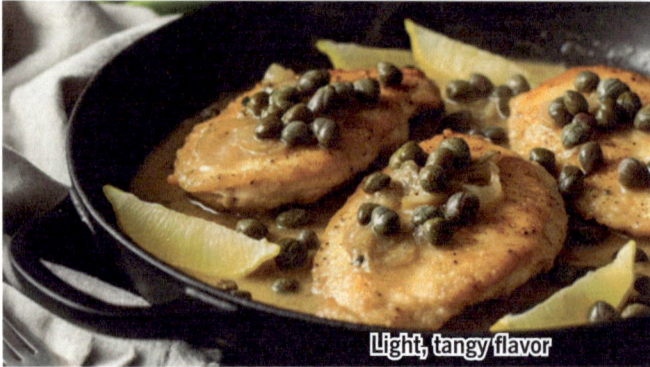

Light, tangy flavor

🍽 4 servings

⏰ Prep Time **10** min

⏳ Cook Time **20** min

Nutritional
Calories: 350 kcal
Protein: 30g
Fats: 15g
Carbs: 15g

Instructions

1. Dredge the chicken breasts in flour, shaking off excess.

2. Heat olive oil in a skillet over medium heat. Cook chicken for 3-4 minutes per side until golden.

3. Add lemon juice, chicken broth, and capers. Simmer for 5 minutes until sauce thickens.

4. Serve with a sprinkle of fresh parsley.

Ingredients

- 4 boneless, skinless chicken breasts
- 1/4 cup all-purpose flour (or gluten-free flour)
- 2 tbsp olive oil
- 1/4 cup fresh lemon juice
- 1/4 cup chicken broth
- 2 tbsp capers, rinsed
- Salt and black pepper to taste
- Fresh parsley for garnish

Ingredient Availability

Found at Walmart, Publix, and Aldi.

Roasted Cauliflower Steaks

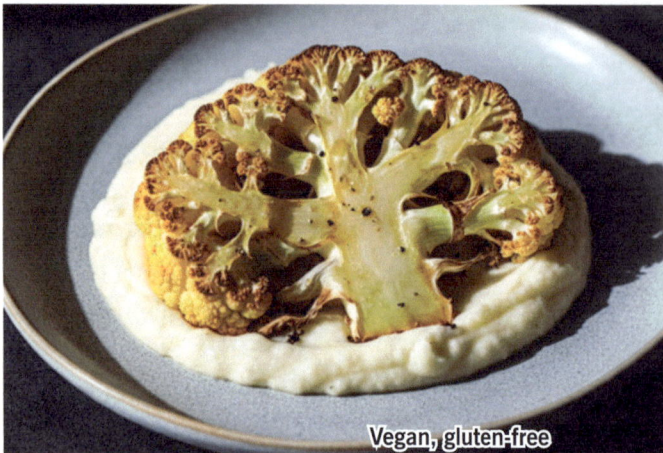

Vegan, gluten-free

🍽 4 servings

⏰ Prep Time **10** min

⏳ Cook Time **25** min

Nutritional
Calories: 150 kcal
Protein: 5g
Fats: 10g
Carbs: 12g

Instructions

1. Preheat oven to 425°F (220°C). Line a baking sheet with parchment paper.

2. Brush both sides of the cauliflower steaks with olive oil. Sprinkle with paprika, garlic powder, salt, and pepper.

3. Roast for 20-25 minutes, flipping halfway through, until golden brown and tender.

4. Garnish with fresh parsley before serving.

Ingredients

- 1 large head of cauliflower, sliced into steaks
- 2 tbsp olive oil
- 1 tsp paprika
- 1/2 tsp garlic powder
- Salt and black pepper to taste
- Fresh parsley for garnish

Ingredient Availability

Available at Aldi, Walmart, and Whole Foods.

Grilled Mahi-Mahi with Mango Salsa

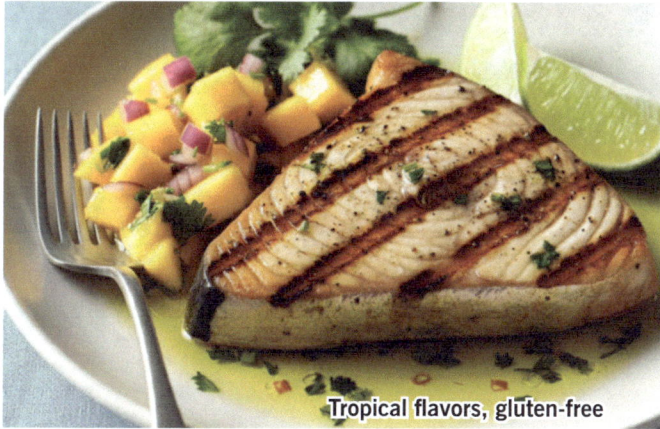

Tropical flavors, gluten-free

4 servings

Prep Time **15** min

Cook Time **10** min

Nutritional
Calories: 320 kcal
Protein: 28g
Fats: 12g
Carbs: 20g

Instructions

1. Preheat grill to medium-high heat. Season mahi-mahi with olive oil, cumin, salt, and pepper.
2. Grill for 3-4 minutes per side until fish flakes easily with a fork.
3. In a bowl, combine mango, red onion, jalapeño, lime juice, and cilantro for the salsa.
4. Serve the grilled mahi-mahi topped with mango salsa.

Ingredients

- 4 mahi-mahi fillets
- 1 tbsp olive oil
- 1/2 tsp cumin
- Salt and black pepper to taste
- 1 ripe mango, diced
- 1/4 cup red onion, diced
- 1 jalapeño, seeded and minced
- 2 tbsp lime juice
- Fresh cilantro for garnish

Ingredient Availability

Found at Target, Publix, and Whole Foods.

Sweet Potato and Black Bean Enchiladas

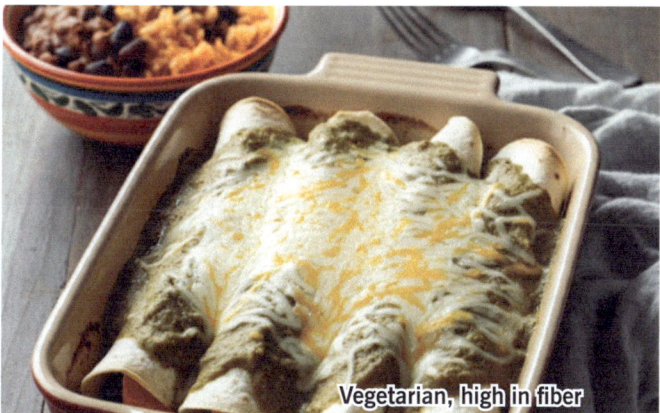

Vegetarian, high in fiber

4 servings

Prep Time **20** min

Cook Time **30** min

Nutritional
Calories: 400 kcal
Protein: 14g
Fats: 15g
Carbs: 50g

Instructions

1. Preheat oven to 375°F (190°C). In a skillet, heat olive oil and cook sweet potatoes until tender, about 10 minutes.
2. Add black beans, cumin, salt, and pepper. Stir well.
3. Fill each tortilla with the sweet potato mixture, roll up, and place in a baking dish.
4. Top with enchilada sauce and cheese. Bake for 20 minutes until bubbly.
5. Garnish with cilantro and serve.

Ingredients

- 2 large sweet potatoes, peeled and diced
- 1 can black beans, drained and rinsed
- 1 cup enchilada sauce
- 8 corn tortillas
- 1/2 cup shredded cheddar cheese
- 1 tbsp olive oil
- 1 tsp cumin
- Salt and black pepper to taste
- Fresh cilantro for garnish

Ingredient Availability

Available at Aldi, Publix, and Walmart.

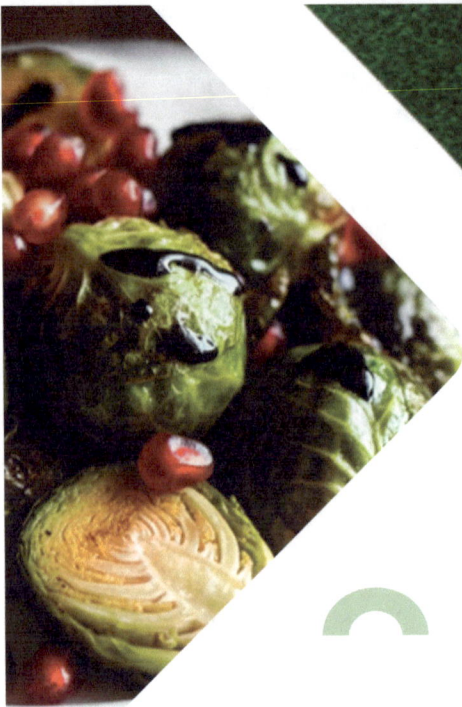

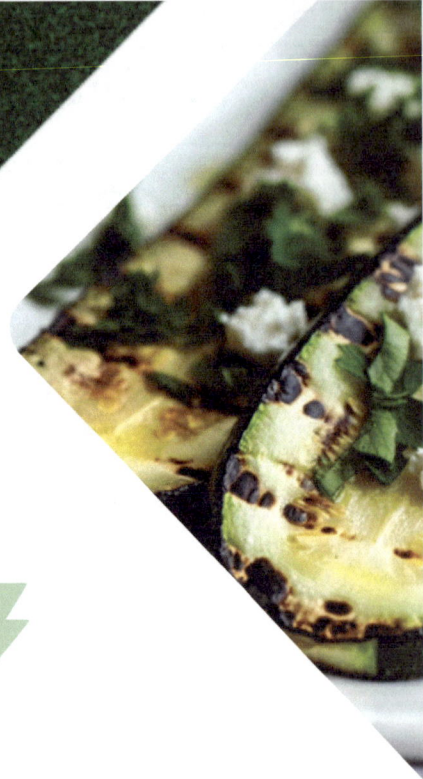

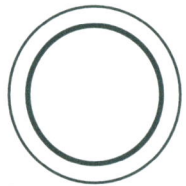

Chapter 6
Sides

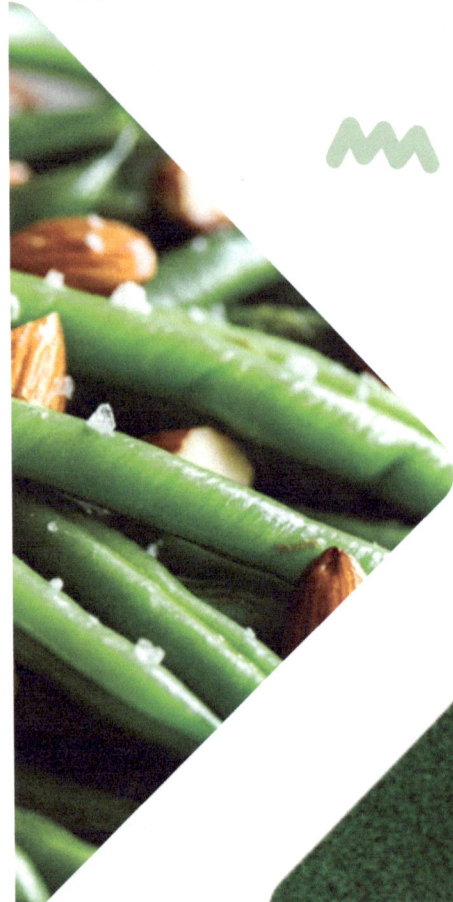

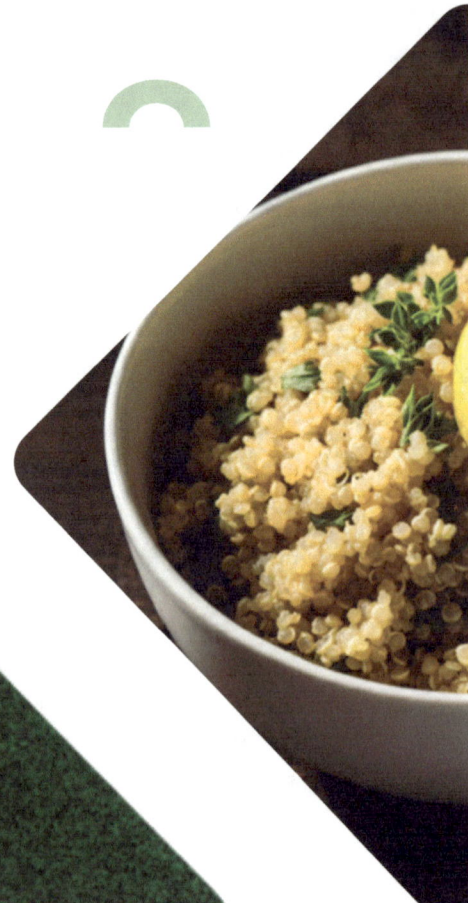

Roasted Brussels Sprouts with Balsamic Glaze

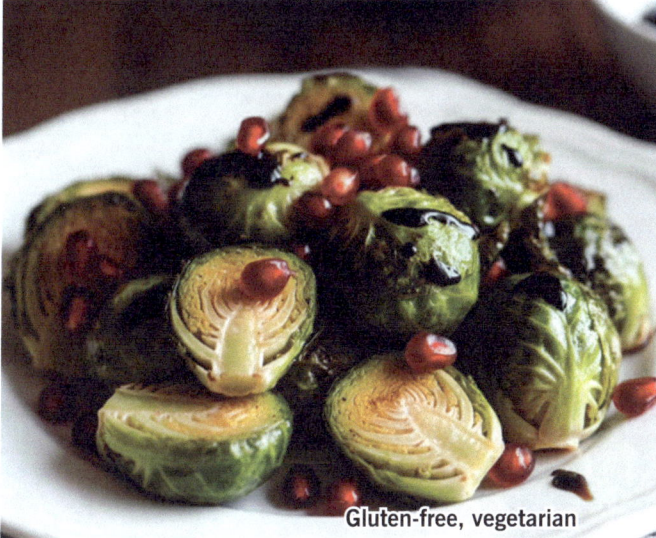

Gluten-free, vegetarian

4 servings

Prep Time **10 min**

Cook Time **25 min**

Nutritional
Calories: 120 kcal
Protein: 4g
Fats: 7g
Carbs: 12g

Instructions

1. Preheat oven to 425°F (220°C). Toss Brussels sprouts with olive oil, salt, and black pepper.

2. Spread on a baking sheet and roast for 20-25 minutes, stirring halfway through.

3. Drizzle with balsamic glaze before serving.

Ingredients

- 1 lb Brussels sprouts, trimmed and halved
- 2 tbsp olive oil
- Salt and black pepper to taste
- 2 tbsp balsamic glaze

Ingredient Availability

Found at Walmart, Aldi, and Whole Foods.

Garlic Mashed Cauliflower

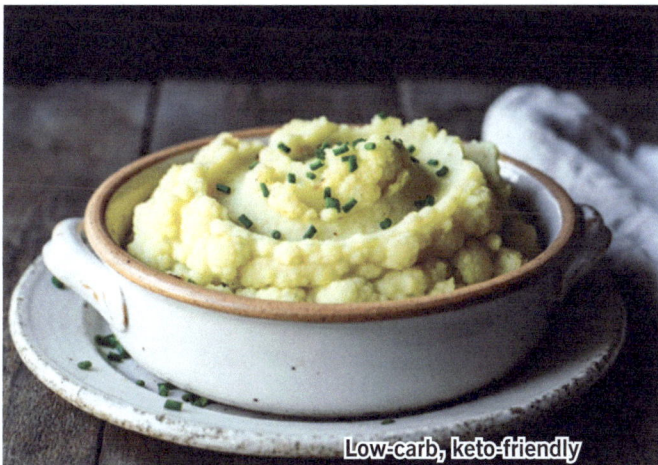

Low-carb, keto-friendly

4 servings

Prep Time **10 min**

Cook Time **15 min**

Nutritional
Calories: 100 kcal
Protein: 3g
Fats: 7g
Carbs: 8g

Instructions

1. Steam cauliflower for 10-12 minutes until tender.

2. Place in a food processor with garlic, butter, and heavy cream. Blend until smooth.

3. Season with salt and black pepper. Garnish with fresh chives before serving.

Ingredients

- 1 large head of cauliflower, chopped
- 2 cloves garlic, minced
- 2 tbsp butter
- 1/4 cup heavy cream
- Salt and black pepper to taste
- Fresh chives for garnish

Ingredient Availability

Available at Publix, Costco, and Whole Foods.

Lemon Herb Quinoa

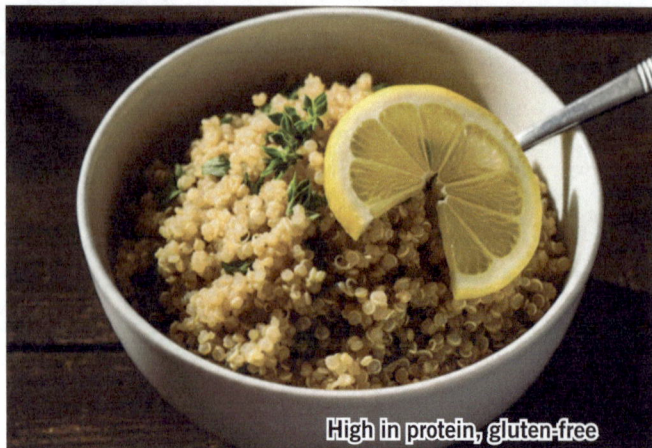
High in protein, gluten-free

4 servings

Prep Time **5 min**

Cook Time **15 min**

Nutritional
Calories: 180 kcal
Protein: 6g
Fats: 8g
Carbs: 24g

Instructions

1. In a pot, combine quinoa and vegetable broth. Bring to a boil, then reduce heat and simmer for 15 minutes or until liquid is absorbed.

2. Fluff with a fork and stir in olive oil, lemon zest, parsley, salt, and black pepper.

3. Serve warm or at room temperature.

Ingredients

- 1 cup quinoa, rinsed
- 2 cups vegetable broth
- 2 tbsp olive oil
- Zest of 1 lemon
- 2 tbsp fresh parsley, chopped
- Salt and black pepper to taste

Ingredient Availability

Found at Whole Foods, Aldi, and Walmart.

Steamed Green Beans with Almonds

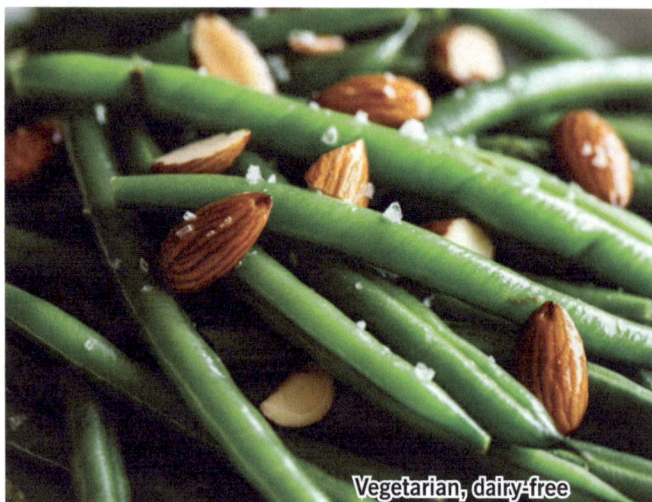
Vegetarian, dairy-free

4 servings

Prep Time **5 min**

Cook Time **10 min**

Nutritional
Calories: 110 kcal
Protein: 3g
Fats: 9g
Carbs: 7g

Instructions

1. Steam green beans for 8-10 minutes until tender-crisp.

2. In a pan, toast almonds over medium heat for 2-3 minutes.

3. Drizzle green beans with olive oil, toss with almonds, and season with salt, black pepper, and lemon juice.

4. Serve immediately.

Ingredients

- 1 lb green beans, trimmed
- 2 tbsp olive oil
- 1/4 cup slivered almonds
- Salt and black pepper to taste
- 1 tbsp lemon juice

Ingredient Availability

Available at Target, Aldi, and Walmart.

Mediterranean Potato Wedges

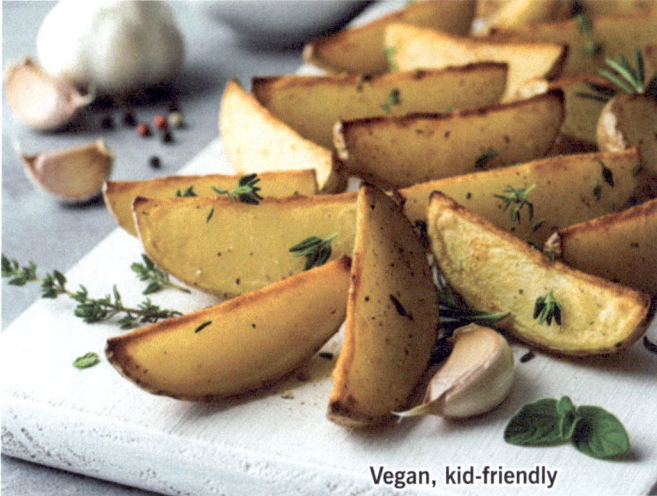

4 servings

Prep Time **10** min

Cook Time **30** min

Nutritional
Calories: 180 kcal
Protein: 4g
Fats: 8g
Carbs: 28g

Instructions

1. Preheat oven to 425°F (220°C). Toss potato wedges with olive oil, oregano, paprika, salt, and black pepper.

2. Spread on a baking sheet and bake for 25-30 minutes, flipping halfway through.

3. Serve warm with your favorite dip.

Vegan, kid-friendly

Ingredients

- 4 medium russet potatoes, cut into wedges
- 3 tbsp olive oil
- 1 tsp dried oregano
- 1/2 tsp paprika
- Salt and black pepper to taste

Ingredient Availability

Found at Aldi, Publix, and Costco.

Grilled Zucchini with Feta

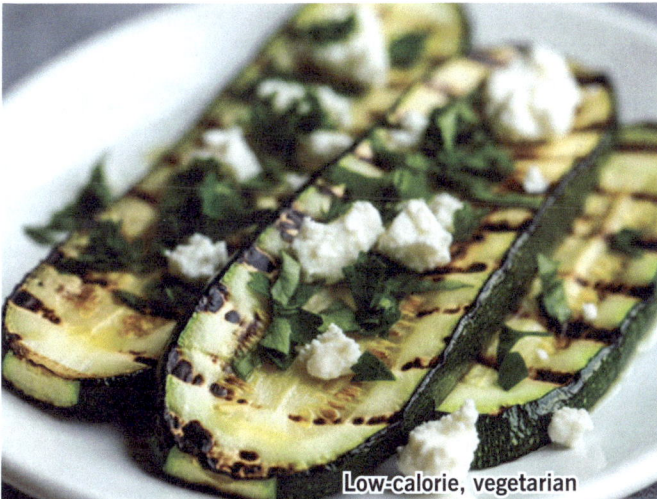

4 servings

Prep Time **5** min

Cook Time **10** min

Nutritional
Calories: 100 kcal
Protein: 4g
Fats: 7g
Carbs: 6g

Instructions

1. Preheat grill or grill pan to medium-high heat.

2. Brush zucchini slices with olive oil, season with salt and black pepper.

3. Grill for 4-5 minutes per side.

4. Sprinkle with feta cheese and fresh dill before serving.

Low-calorie, vegetarian

Ingredients

- 3 medium zucchinis, sliced lengthwise
- 2 tbsp olive oil
- Salt and black pepper to taste
- 1/4 cup crumbled feta cheese
- 1 tbsp fresh dill, chopped

Ingredient Availability

Found at Walmart, Aldi, and Whole Foods.

Garlic Roasted Carrots

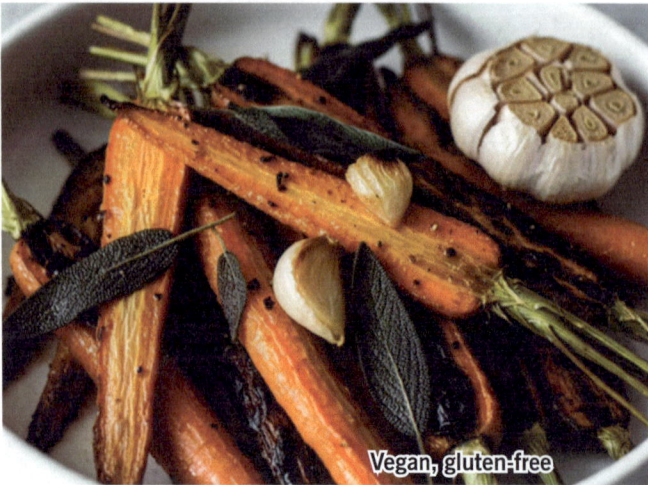

Vegan, gluten-free

4 servings

Prep Time **5** min

Cook Time **25** min

Nutritional
Calories: 120 kcal
Protein: 2g
Fats: 7g
Carbs: 13g

Instructions

1. Preheat oven to 425°F (220°C). In a bowl, toss carrots with olive oil, garlic, salt, black pepper, and thyme.

2. Spread carrots on a baking sheet and roast for 20-25 minutes, stirring halfway through.

3. Serve warm as a side dish.

Ingredients

- 1 lb carrots, peeled and cut into sticks
- 2 tbsp olive oil
- 3 cloves garlic, minced
- Salt and black pepper to taste
- 1 tsp dried thyme

Ingredient Availability

Found at Aldi, Publix, and Walmart.

Cucumber and Tomato Salad

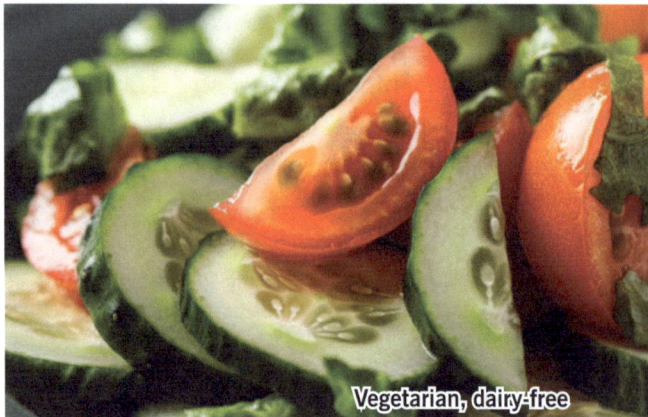

Vegetarian, dairy-free

4 servings

Prep Time **10** min

Cook Time **0** min

Nutritional
Calories: 80 kcal
Protein: 2g
Fats: 5g
Carbs: 9g

Instructions

1. In a large bowl, combine cucumbers, tomatoes, and red onion.

2. Drizzle with olive oil and red wine vinegar. Season with salt and black pepper.

3. Toss gently and sprinkle with fresh parsley before serving.

Ingredients

- 2 medium cucumbers, diced
- 3 ripe tomatoes, diced
- 1/4 red onion, thinly sliced
- 2 tbsp olive oil
- 1 tbsp red wine vinegar
- Salt and black pepper to taste
- 1 tbsp fresh parsley, chopped

Ingredient Availability

Available at Walmart, Target, and Whole Foods.

Spinach and Feta Stuffed Mushrooms

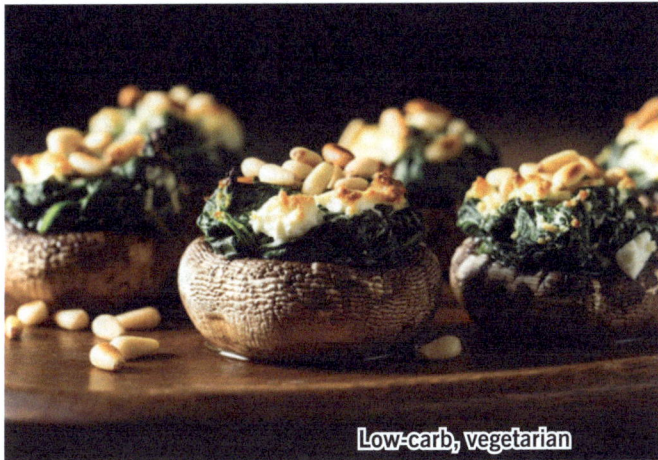

4 servings

Prep Time **10** min

Cook Time **15** min

Nutritional
Calories: 90 kcal
Protein: 4g
Fats: 6g
Carbs: 4g

Low-carb, vegetarian

Instructions

1. Preheat oven to 400°F (200°C). Place mushroom caps on a baking sheet.

2. In a pan, sauté spinach and garlic in olive oil until wilted. Remove from heat and stir in feta cheese, salt, and black pepper.

3. Spoon the mixture into the mushroom caps and bake for 12-15 minutes.

4. Serve warm as an appetizer or side dish.

Ingredients

- 12 large white mushrooms, stems removed
- 1 cup fresh spinach, chopped
- 1/2 cup feta cheese, crumbled
- 1 clove garlic, minced
- 1 tbsp olive oil
- Salt and black pepper to taste

Ingredient Availability

Found at Aldi, Publix, and Whole Foods.

Cauliflower Rice Pilaf

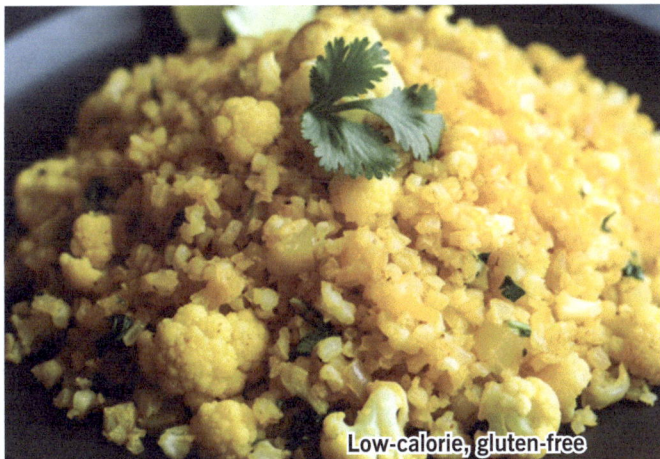

4 servings

Prep Time **10** min

Cook Time **10** min

Nutritional
Calories: 100 kcal
Protein: 3g
Fats: 7g
Carbs: 7g

Low-calorie, gluten-free

Instructions

1. In a pan, heat olive oil over medium heat. Sauté onion for 3-4 minutes.

2. Add riced cauliflower, cumin, salt, and black pepper. Cook for 5-6 minutes.

3. Stir in slivered almonds and cook for another 2 minutes.

4. Serve as a side dish.

Ingredients

- 1 head of cauliflower, riced
- 1/4 cup chopped onion
- 1/4 cup slivered almonds
- 1 tbsp olive oil
- 1/2 tsp cumin
- Salt and black pepper to taste

Ingredient Availability

Found at Costco, Whole Foods, and Walmart.

Oven-Baked Sweet Potato Fries

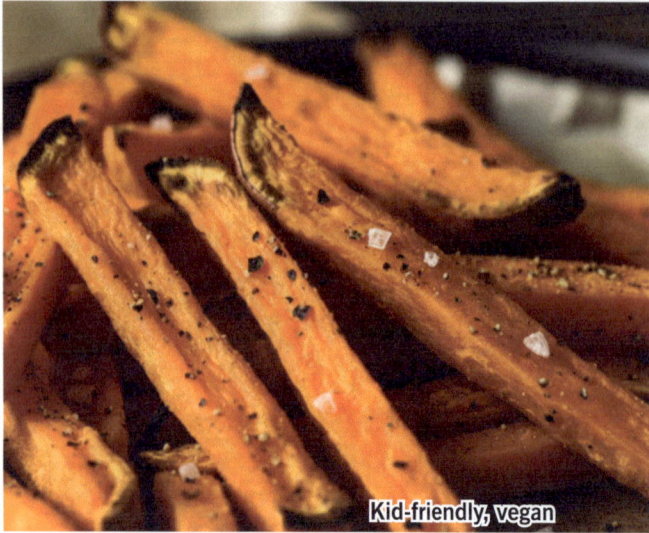

Kid-friendly, vegan

4 servings

Prep Time **10 min**

Cook Time **25 min**

Nutritional
Calories: 160 kcal
Protein: 2g
Fats: 7g
Carbs: 22g

Instructions

1. Preheat oven to 425°F (220°C). Toss sweet potato fries with olive oil, paprika, salt, and black pepper.

2. Spread on a baking sheet and bake for 25 minutes, flipping halfway.

3. Serve with your favorite dipping sauce.

Ingredients

- 2 large sweet potatoes, cut into fries
- 2 tbsp olive oil
- 1/2 tsp paprika
- Salt and black pepper to taste

Ingredient Availability

Available at Aldi, Target, and Whole Foods.

Bulgur with Dried Cranberries

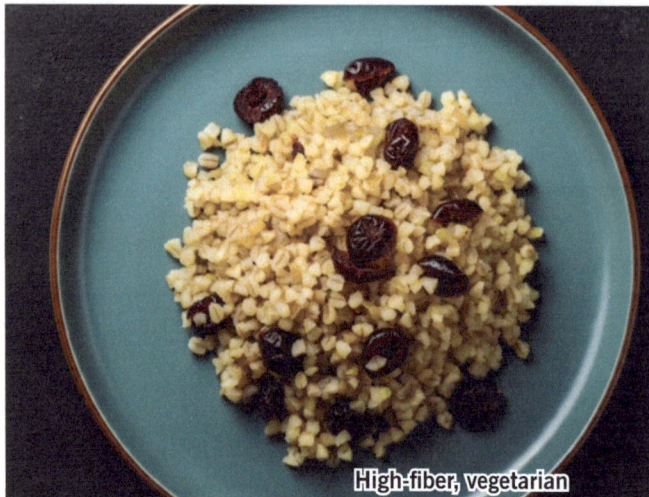

High-fiber, vegetarian

4 servings

Prep Time **5 min**

Cook Time **15 min**

Nutritional
Calories: 170 kcal
Protein: 5g
Fats: 4g
Carbs: 28g

Instructions

1. In a pot, combine bulgur wheat and vegetable broth. Bring to a boil, then reduce heat and simmer for 15 minutes.

2. Stir in dried cranberries, olive oil, salt, and black pepper.

3. Serve warm or at room temperature.

Ingredients

- 1 cup bulgur wheat
- 2 cups vegetable broth
- 1/4 cup dried cranberries
- 1 tbsp olive oil
- Salt and black pepper to taste

Ingredient Availability

Found at Whole Foods, Walmart, and Publix.

Roasted Beets with Goat Cheese

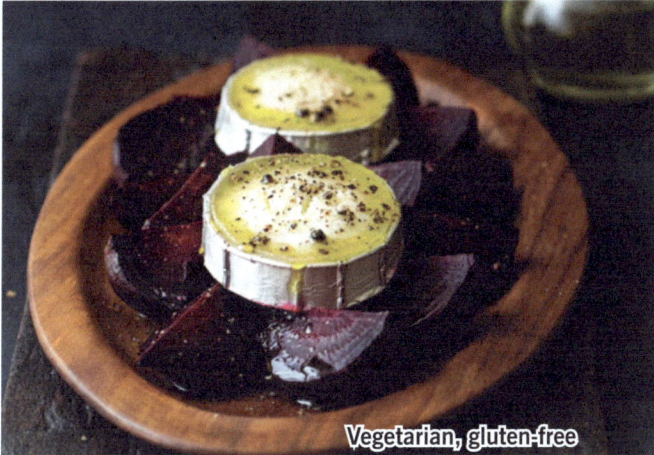

4 servings

Prep Time **10** min

Cook Time **45** min

Nutritional
Calories: 150 kcal
Protein: 4g
Fats: 7g
Carbs: 16g

Vegetarian, gluten-free

Instructions

1. Preheat oven to 400°F (200°C). Wrap each beet in foil and roast for 40-45 minutes or until tender.

2. Let cool, peel, and slice beets into wedges.

3. Arrange beet slices on a plate, drizzle with olive oil and balsamic vinegar, and season with salt and black pepper.

4. Top with crumbled goat cheese and garnish with fresh parsley.

Ingredients

- 4 medium beets, washed and trimmed
- 2 tbsp olive oil
- Salt and black pepper to taste
- 1/4 cup goat cheese, crumbled
- 1 tbsp balsamic vinegar
- Fresh parsley for garnish

Ingredient Availability

Found at Aldi, Whole Foods, and Publix.

Warm Lentil Salad with Tomatoes

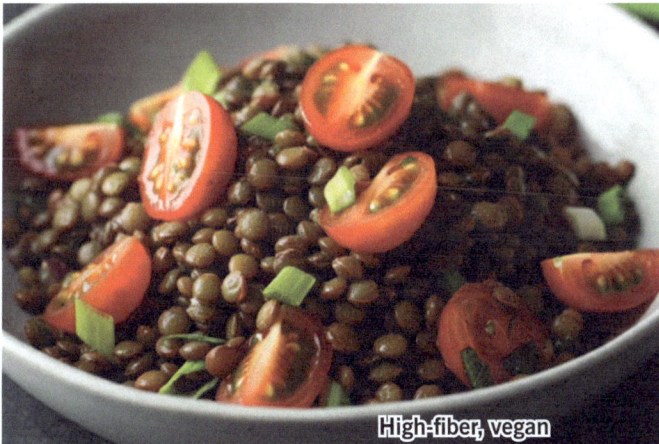

4 servings

Prep Time **10** min

Cook Time **20** min

Nutritional
Calories: 180 kcal
Protein: 9g
Fats: 8g
Carbs: 22g

High-fiber, vegan

Instructions

1. In a pot, cook lentils in vegetable broth for 20 minutes or until tender. Drain and let cool slightly.

2. In a large bowl, combine lentils, cherry tomatoes, and red onion.

3. Drizzle with olive oil and red wine vinegar, season with salt and black pepper, and toss.

4. Garnish with fresh dill before serving warm.

Ingredients

- 1 cup green lentils, rinsed
- 2 cups vegetable broth
- 1 cup cherry tomatoes, halved
- 1/4 cup red onion, diced
- 2 tbsp olive oil
- 1 tbsp red wine vinegar
- Salt and black pepper to taste
- 1 tbsp fresh dill, chopped

Ingredient Availability

Available at Walmart, Target, and Whole Foods.

Baked Broccoli with Parmesan

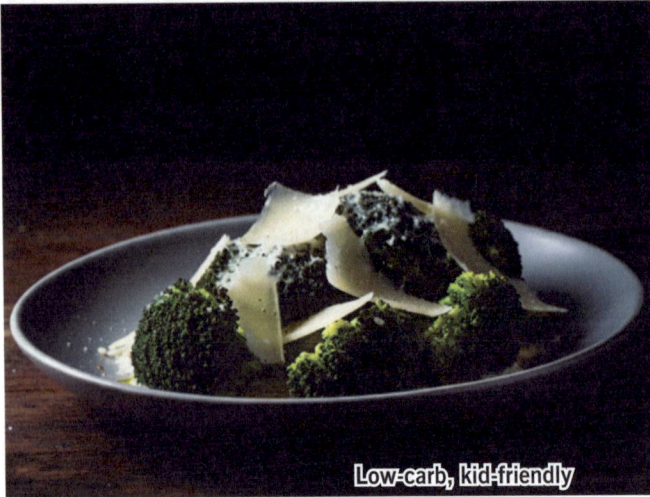

Low-carb, kid-friendly

4 servings

Prep Time **5** min

Cook Time **20** min

Nutritional
Calories: 130 kcal
Protein: 5g
Fats: 9g
Carbs: 9g

Instructions

1. Preheat oven to 425°F (220°C). Toss broccoli florets with olive oil, garlic powder, salt, and black pepper.

2. Spread on a baking sheet and bake for 15 minutes.

3. Sprinkle with Parmesan cheese and bake for another 5 minutes.

4. Serve immediately

Ingredients

- 2 heads of broccoli, cut into florets
- 2 tbsp olive oil
- 1/4 cup grated Parmesan cheese
- Salt and black pepper to taste
- 1/2 tsp garlic powder

Ingredient Availability

Found at Aldi, Costco, and Publix.

Ratatouille

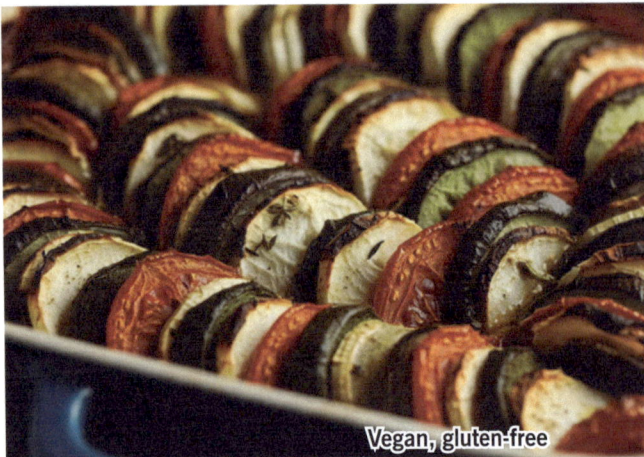

Vegan, gluten-free

4 servings

Prep Time **15** min

Cook Time **45** min

Nutritional
Calories: 160 kcal
Protein: 3g
Fats: 11g
Carbs: 15g

Instructions

1. Preheat oven to 375°F (190°C). In a large baking dish, combine eggplant, zucchini, bell pepper, tomatoes, and onion.

2. Drizzle with olive oil, add minced garlic, thyme, salt, and black pepper. Mix well.

3. Bake for 45 minutes, stirring halfway through.

4. Garnish with fresh basil before serving.

Ingredients

- 1 eggplant, diced
- 2 zucchinis, sliced
- 1 bell pepper, diced
- 2 tomatoes, chopped
- 1/2 onion, chopped
- 3 tbsp olive oil
- 2 cloves garlic, minced
- 1 tsp dried thyme
- Salt and black pepper to taste
- Fresh basil for garnish

Ingredient Availability

Available at Whole Foods, Publix, and Walmart

Sautéed Kale with Lemon

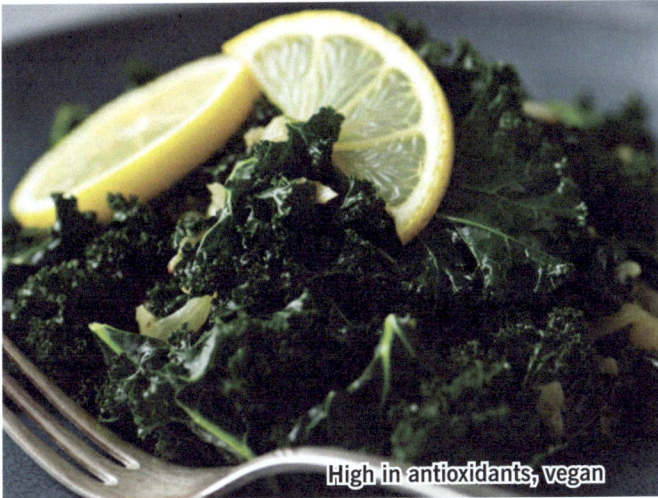

High in antioxidants, vegan

4 servings

Prep Time **5 min**

Cook Time **10 min**

Nutritional
Calories: 80 kcal
Protein: 2g
Fats: 5g
Carbs: 8g

Instructions

1. Heat olive oil in a large skillet over medium heat. Add garlic and sauté for 1 minute.

2. Add kale and cook for 5-7 minutes, until wilted.

3. Drizzle with lemon juice, season with salt and black pepper, and serve warm.

Ingredients

- 1 bunch kale, chopped
- 1 tbsp olive oil
- 1 clove garlic, minced
- 1 tbsp lemon juice
- Salt and black pepper to taste

Ingredient Availability

Found at Aldi, Whole Foods, and Walmart.

Caponata with Eggplant

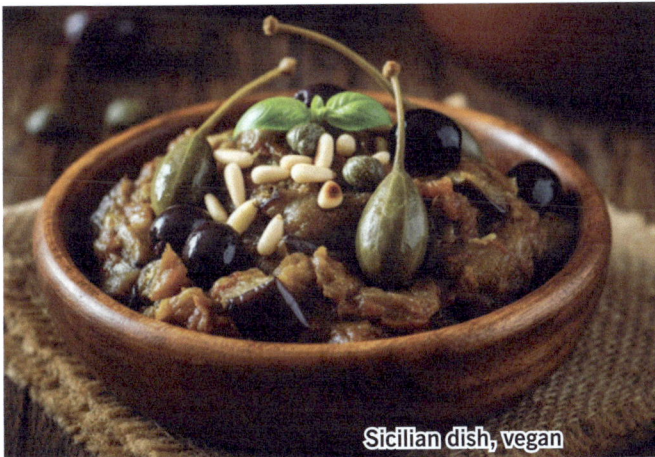

Sicilian dish, vegan

4 servings

Prep Time **15 min**

Cook Time **30 min**

Nutritional
Calories: 200 kcal
Protein: 2g
Fats: 14g
Carbs: 16g

Instructions

1. Heat half the olive oil in a large pan over medium heat. Add eggplant and sauté for 10 minutes until golden. Remove from pan.

2. In the same pan, add remaining olive oil and sauté celery for 5 minutes. Add olives, capers, tomato paste, and vinegar. Mix well.

3. Return eggplant to the pan, season with salt and black pepper, and cook for an additional 10 minutes.

4. Serve warm or at room temperature.

Ingredients

- 1/2 cup diced celery
- 1/4 cup green olives, chopped
- 2 tbsp capers, rinsed
- 1/4 cup tomato paste
- 2 tbsp red wine vinegar
- Salt and black pepper to taste

Ingredient Availability

Available at Aldi, Publix, and Whole Foods.

Moroccan-Spiced Carrots

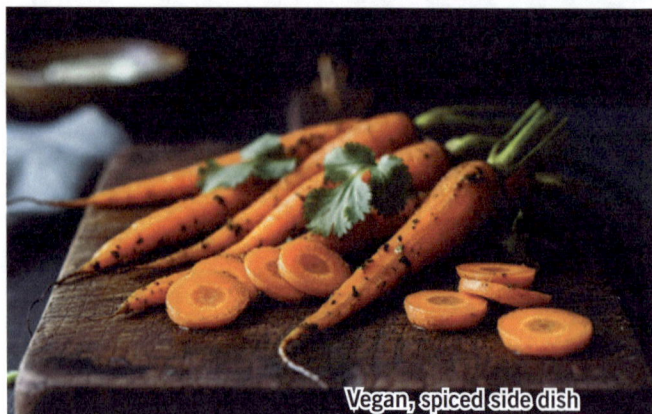

Vegan, spiced side dish

4 servings

Prep Time **5** min

Cook Time **15** min

Nutritional
Calories: 110 kcal
Protein: 1g
Fats: 7g
Carbs: 10g

Instructions

1. Preheat oven to 400°F (200°C). Toss carrots with olive oil, cumin, cinnamon, paprika, salt, and black pepper.

2. Spread carrots on a baking sheet and roast for 15 minutes or until tender.

3. Garnish with chopped cilantro before serving, if desired.

Ingredients

- 1 lb carrots, peeled and sliced
- 2 tbsp olive oil
- 1/2 tsp ground cumin
- 1/2 tsp ground cinnamon
- 1/4 tsp paprika
- Salt and black pepper to taste
- 1 tbsp fresh cilantro, chopped (optional)

Ingredient Availability

Available at Walmart, Aldi, and Whole Foods.

Herb Roasted Potatoes

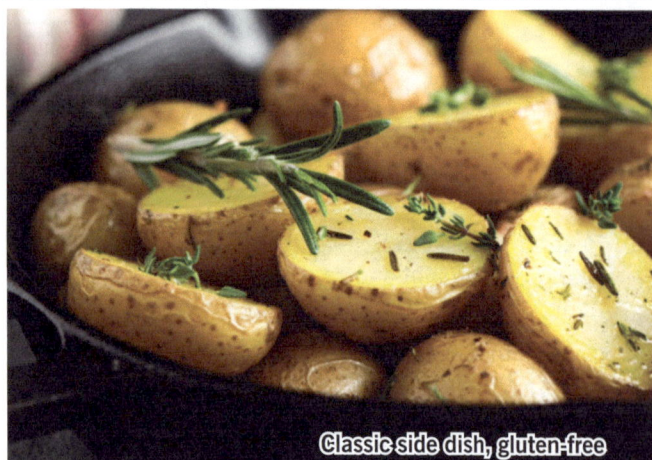

Classic side dish, gluten-free

4 servings

Prep Time **10** min

Cook Time **30** min

Nutritional
Calories: 180 kcal
Protein: 3g
Fats: 9g
Carbs: 22g

Instructions

1. Preheat oven to 425°F (220°C). Toss potatoes with olive oil, rosemary, garlic powder, salt, and black pepper in a large bowl.

2. Spread potatoes on a baking sheet in a single layer.

3. Roast for 30 minutes or until golden brown and crispy.

4. Garnish with fresh parsley before serving.

Ingredients

- 1.5 lbs baby potatoes, halved
- 3 tbsp olive oil
- 1 tbsp fresh rosemary, chopped
- 1 tsp garlic powder
- Salt and black pepper to taste
- Fresh parsley for garnish

Ingredient Availability

Found at Aldi, Publix, and Walmart.

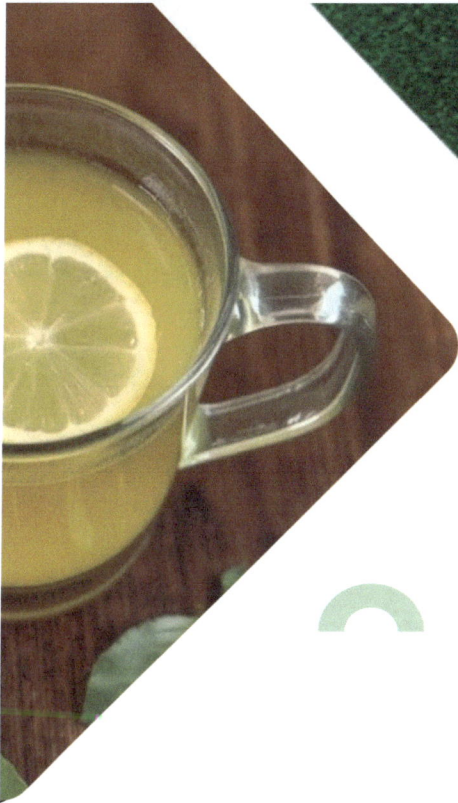

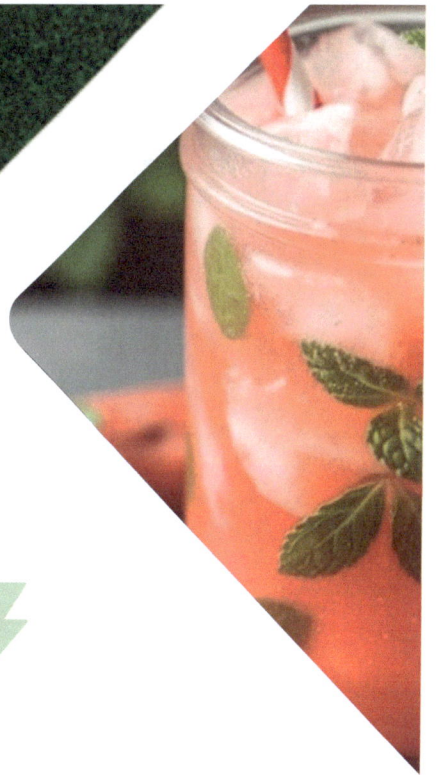

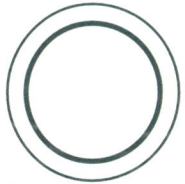

Chapter 7
Drinks and Smoothies

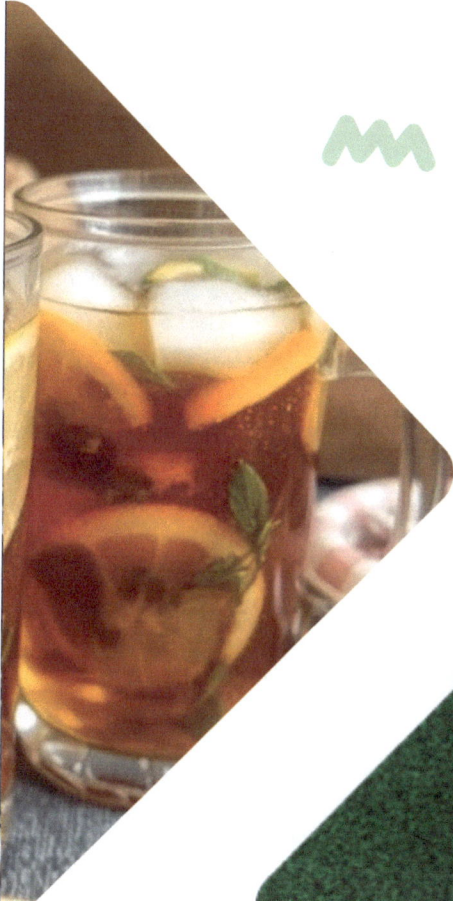

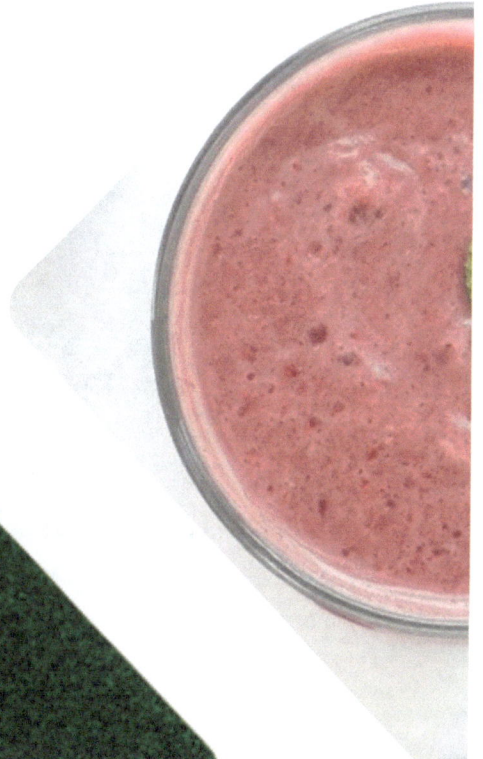

Watermelon Mint Cooler

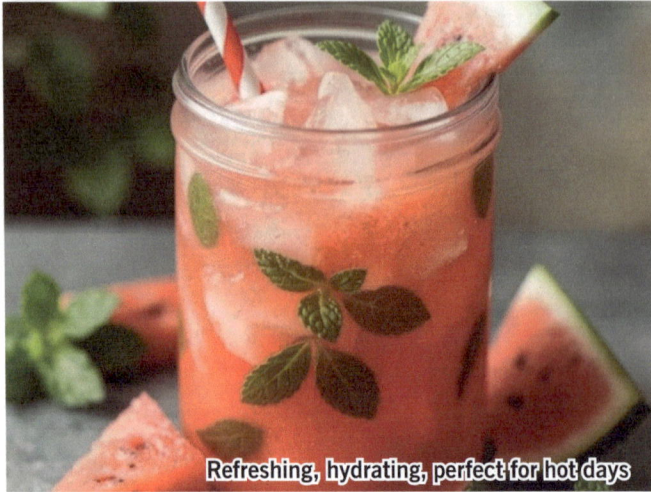

4 servings

Prep Time **10** min

Cook Time **0** min

Nutritional
Calories: 60 kcal
Protein: 1g
Fats: 0g
Carbs: 15g

Instructions

1. Blend the watermelon, mint leaves, lime juice, and honey (if using) until smooth.
2. Strain the mixture through a fine sieve into a pitcher.
3. Serve over ice cubes and garnish with mint leaves.

Refreshing, hydrating, perfect for hot days

Ingredients

- 4 cups watermelon, cubed and chilled
- 1/4 cup fresh mint leaves
- 2 tbsp lime juice
- 1 tbsp honey (optional)
- Ice cubes for serving

Ingredient Availability
Found at Walmart and Target.

Green Tea with Ginger and Lemon

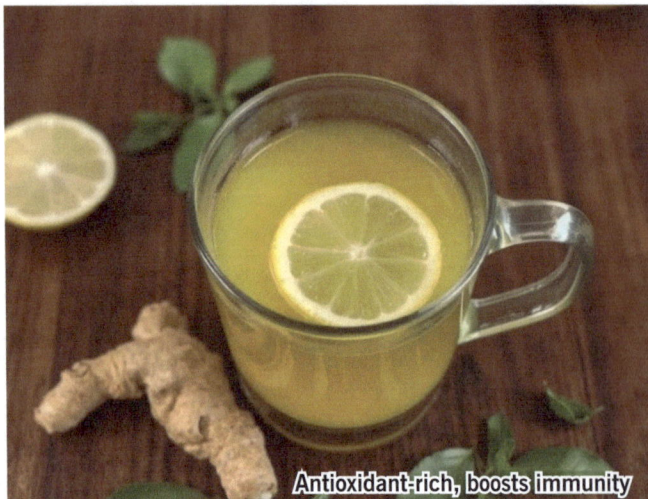

4 servings

Prep Time **5** min

Cook Time **5** min

Nutritional
Calories: 10 kcal
Protein: 0g
Fats: 0g
Carbs: 3g

Instructions

1. Bring water and ginger slices to a boil in a saucepan. Simmer for 5 minutes.
2. Remove from heat, add green tea bags, and steep for 3-4 minutes.
3. Strain into cups, add lemon slices, and sweeten with honey if desired

Antioxidant-rich, boosts immunity

Ingredients

- 4 cups water
- 2-inch piece of fresh ginger, sliced
- 4 green tea bags
- 1 lemon, sliced
- Honey to taste (optional)

Ingredient Availability
Available at Aldi and Publix.

Berry Blast Smoothie

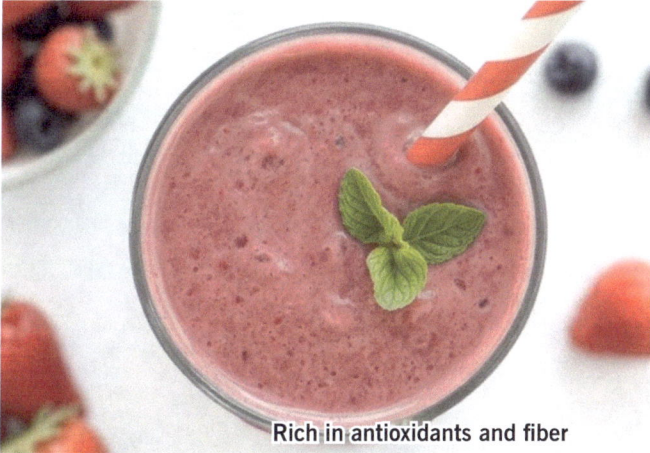

🍽️ 2 servings

⏰ Prep Time **5** min

⏳ Cook Time **0** min

Nutritional
Calories: 150 kcal
Protein: 8g
Fats: 3g
Carbs: 26g

Instructions

1. Blend all ingredients until smooth.
2. Pour into glasses and serve chilled.

Rich in antioxidants and fiber

Ingredients

- 1 cup mixed frozen berries (strawberries, blueberries, raspberries)
- 1/2 cup plain Greek yogurt
- 1/2 cup almond milk
- 1 tbsp honey (optional)
- 1 tbsp chia seeds

Ingredient Availability

Available at Costco and Whole Foods.

Iced Citrus Herbal Tea

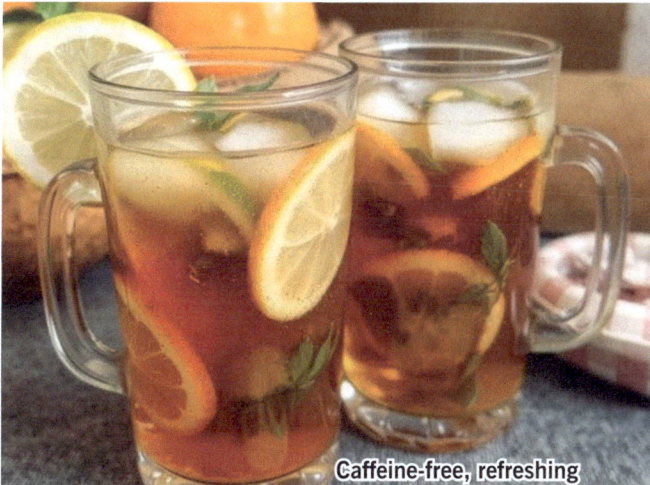

🍽️ 4 servings

⏰ Prep Time **5** min

⏳ Cook Time **10** min

Nutritional
Calories: 5 kcal
Protein: 0g
Fats: 0g
Carbs: 1g

Instructions

1. Bring water to a boil and steep the tea bags for 5-7 minutes.
2. Let the tea cool to room temperature, then refrigerate for 30 minutes.
3. Serve over ice with orange and lemon slices.

Caffeine-free, refreshing

Ingredients

- 4 cups water
- 4 herbal tea bags (citrus flavor)
- 1 orange, sliced
- 1 lemon, sliced
- Ice cubes for serving

Ingredient Availability

Available at Harris Teeter and Whole Foods.

Mango Pineapple Smoothie

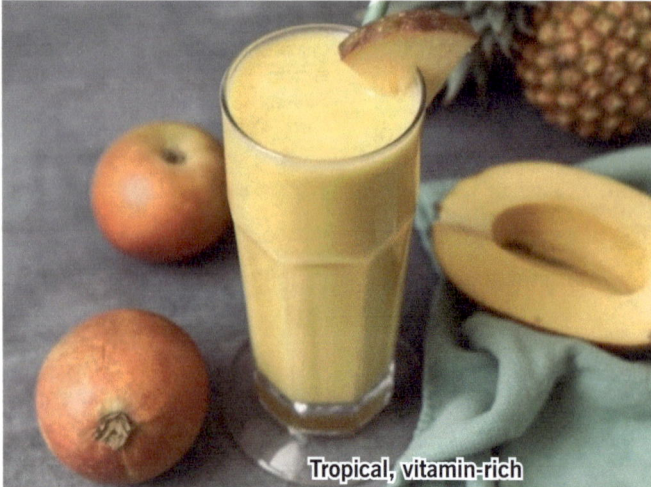

Tropical, vitamin-rich

2 servings

Prep Time **5** min

Cook Time **0** min

Nutritional
Calories: 180 kcal
Protein: 8g
Fats: 2g
Carbs: 35g

Instructions

1. Blend all ingredients until smooth.
2. Serve immediately in chilled glasses.

Ingredients

- 1 cup frozen mango chunks
- 1/2 cup frozen pineapple chunks
- 1/2 cup coconut water
- 1/2 cup plain Greek yogurt
- 1 tbsp honey (optional)

Ingredient Availability

Found at Target and Aldi.

Lemon Cucumber Water

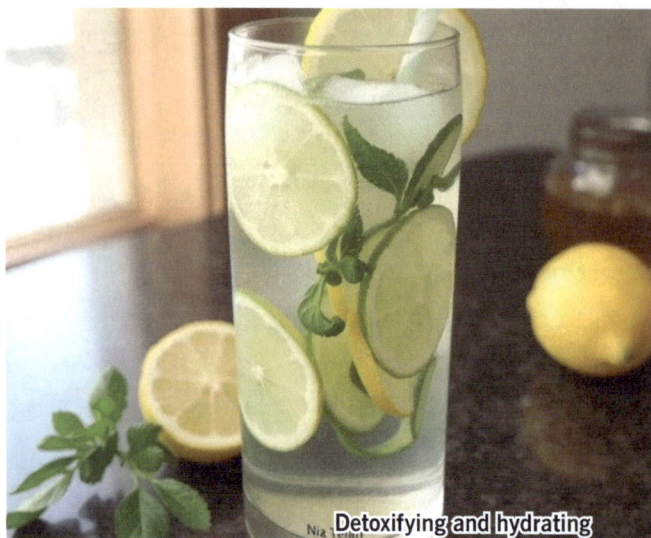

Detoxifying and hydrating

4 servings

Prep Time **5** min

Cook Time **0** min

Nutritional
Calories: 0 kcal
Protein: 0g
Fats: 0g
Carbs: 0g

Instructions

1. Combine water, cucumber slices, lemon slices, and mint leaves in a pitcher.
2. Chill in the refrigerator for at least 1 hour before serving.

Ingredients

- 4 cups cold water
- 1 cucumber, thinly sliced
- 1 lemon, thinly sliced
- Fresh mint leaves (optional)

Ingredient Availability

Available at Walmart and Publix.

Pomegranate and Basil Infused Water

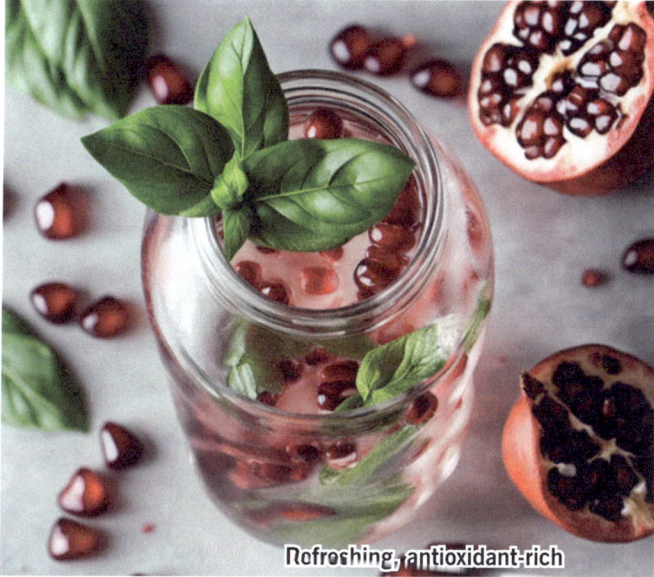

🍽 2 servings

⏱ Prep Time **5** min

⏳ Cook Time **0** min

Nutritional
Calories: 5 kcal
Protein: 0g
Fats: 0g
Carbs: 1g

Refreshing, antioxidant-rich

Instructions

1. Combine water, pomegranate seeds, and basil leaves in a pitcher.
2. Refrigerate for at least 1 hour to infuse the flavors.
3. Serve over ice.

Ingredients

- 4 cups water
- 1/2 cup pomegranate seeds
- Fresh basil leaves

Ingredient Availability

Found at Whole Foods and Costco.

Almond Milk Smoothie with Dates

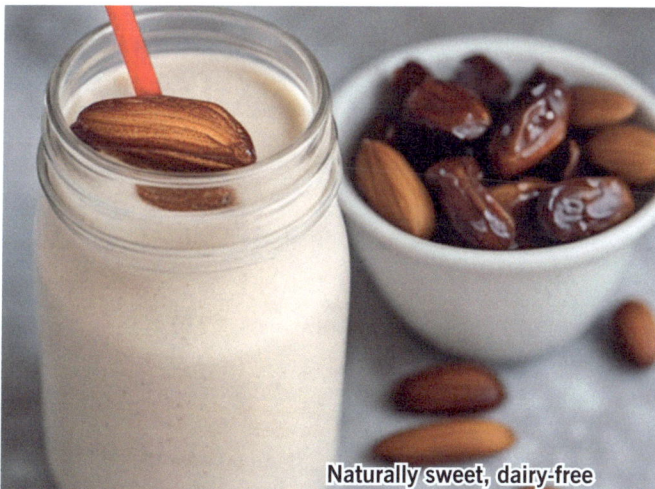

🍽 2 servings

⏱ Prep Time **5** min

⏳ Cook Time **10** min

Nutritional
Calories: 120 kcal
Protein: 2g
Fats: 2g
Carbs: 25g

Naturally sweet, dairy-free

Instructions

1. Blend all ingredients until smooth.
2. Pour into glasses and serve chilled.

Ingredients

- 1 cup unsweetened almond milk
- 4 dates, pitted
- 1/2 banana
- 1/2 tsp vanilla extract
- Ice cubes for serving

Ingredient Availability

Available at Publix and Harris Teeter.

Chia Seed Lemonade

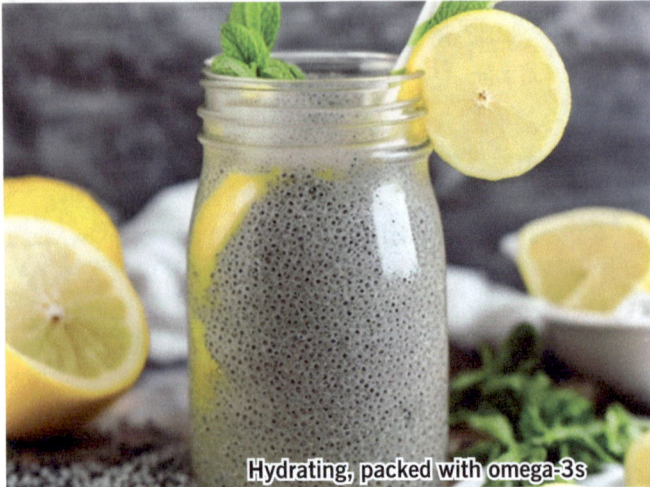

Hydrating, packed with omega-3s

🍴 4 servings

Prep Time **5** min

Cook Time **0** min

Nutritional
Calories: 40 kcal
Protein: 1g
Fats: 1g
Carbs: 9g

Instructions

1. Mix water, lemon juice, and honey in a pitcher.
2. Stir in chia seeds and let sit for 10 minutes, stirring occasionally.
3. Serve over ice.

Ingredients

- 4 cups water
- Juice of 2 lemons
- 2 tbsp chia seeds
- 1 tbsp honey (optional)
- Ice cubes for serving

Ingredient Availability

Available at Walmart and Aldi.

Peach and Mint Iced Tea

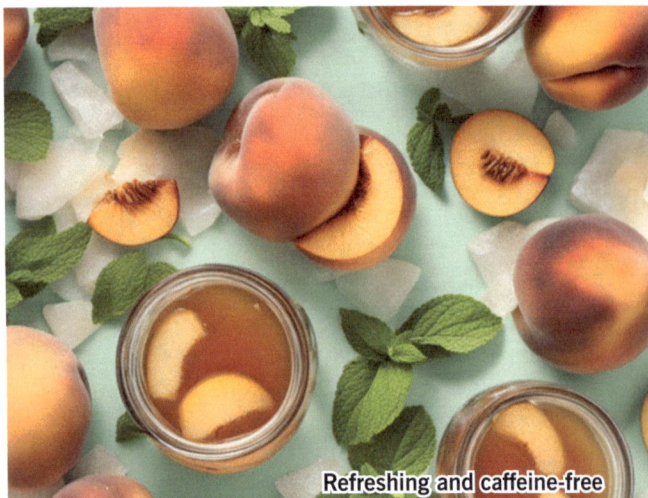

Refreshing and caffeine-free

🍴 4 servings

Prep Time **5** min

Brew Time **15** min

Nutritional
Calories: 10 kcal
Protein: 0g
Fats: 0g
Carbs: 2g

Instructions

1. Boil water and steep the tea bags for 10 minutes.
2. Remove tea bags and let cool to room temperature.
3. Add peach slices and mint leaves. Chill in the refrigerator for 1 hour.
4. Serve over ice.

Ingredients

- 4 cups water
- 2 peach-flavored tea bags
- 1 peach, sliced
- Fresh mint leaves
- Ice cubes for serving

Ingredient Availability

Available at Target and Aldi.

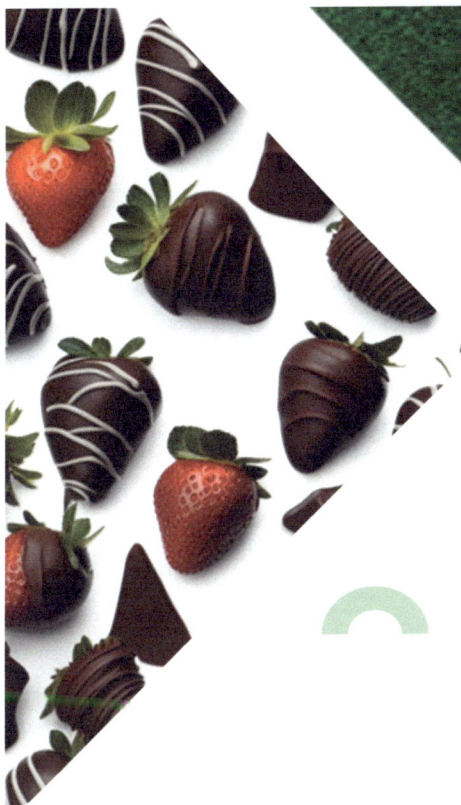

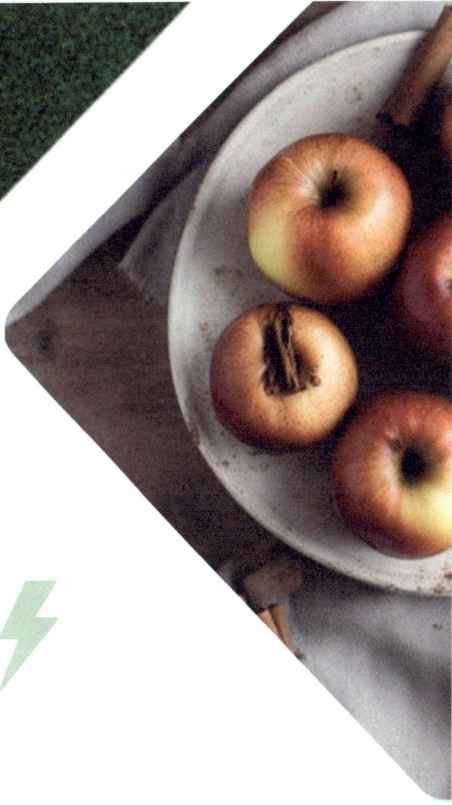

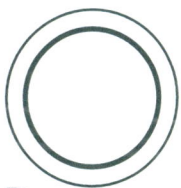

Chapter 8
Desserts

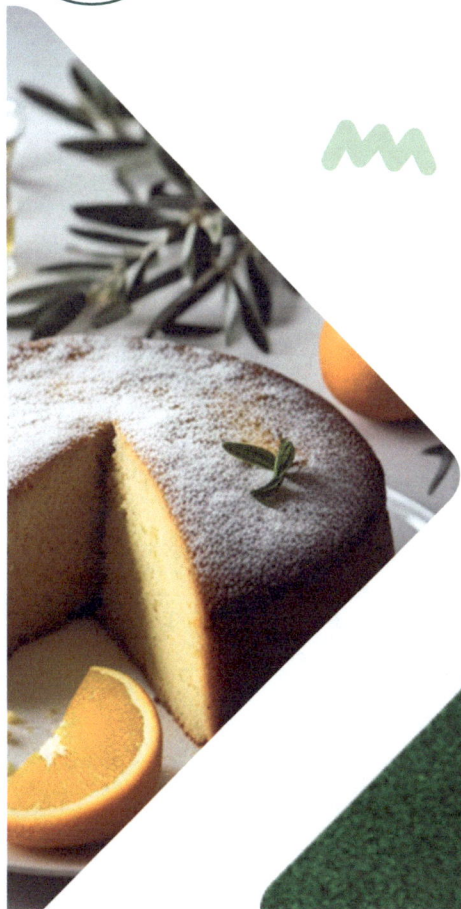

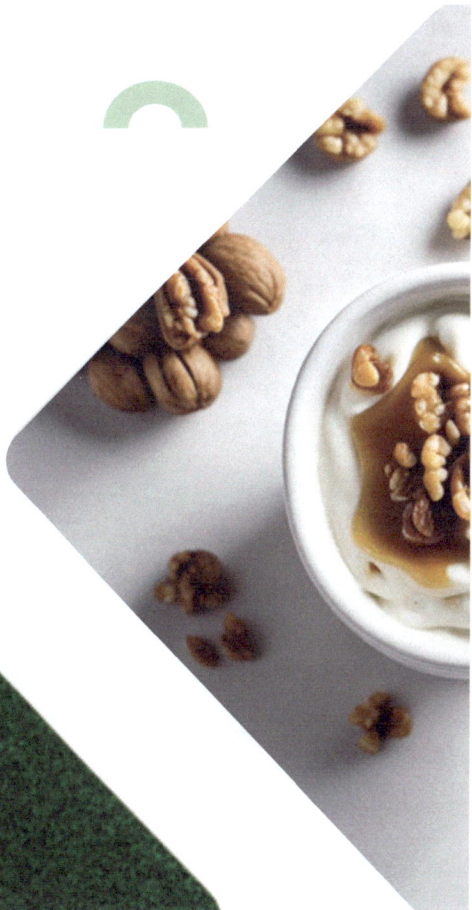

Greek Yogurt with Honey and Walnuts

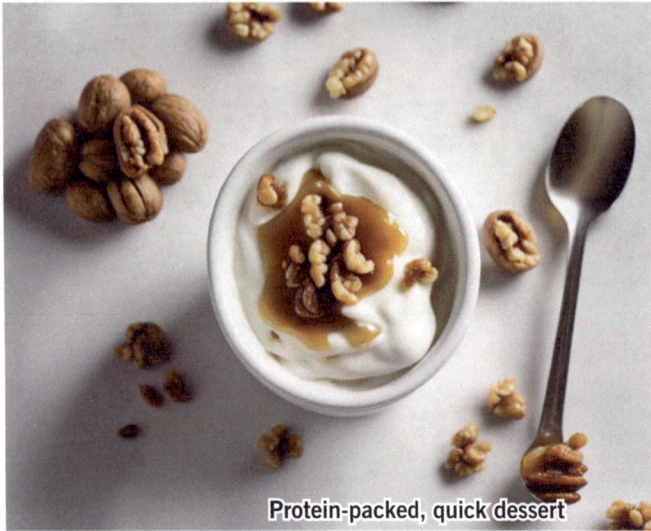

🍽 2 servings

⏱ Prep Time **5** min

⏳ Cook Time **0** min

Nutritional
Calories: 220 kcal
Protein: 10g
Fats: 10g
Carbs: 24g

Instructions

1. Divide the Greek yogurt between two serving bowls.
2. Drizzle each with honey and sprinkle with chopped walnuts.
3. Add a pinch of cinnamon if desired and serve

Protein-packed, quick dessert

Ingredients

- 1 cup Greek yogurt
- 2 tbsp honey
- 1/4 cup walnuts, chopped
- A pinch of cinnamon (optional)

Ingredient Availability

Found at Walmart and Whole Foods.

Olive Oil and Orange Cake

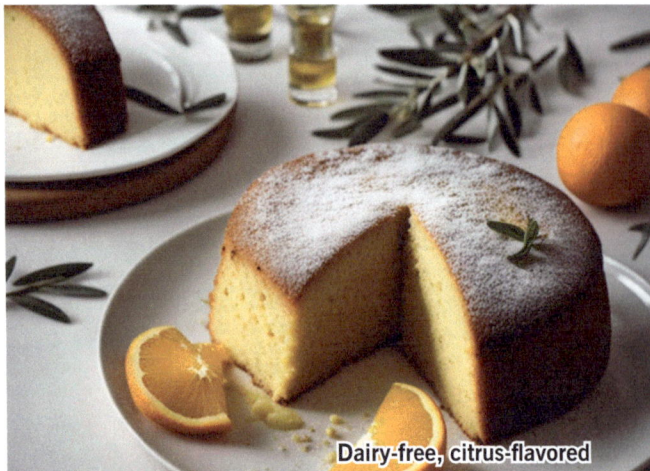

🍽 8 servings

⏱ Prep Time **15** min

⏳ Cook Time **35** min

Nutritional
Calories: 280 kcal
Protein: 4g
Fats: 14g
Carbs: 35g

Instructions

1. Preheat oven to 350°F (175°C). Grease an 8-inch round cake pan.
2. In a bowl, mix olive oil and sugar until combined. Add eggs one at a time, beating well after each.
3. Stir in orange zest and juice.
4. Gradually fold in flour, baking powder, and salt until just combined.
5. Pour batter into the pan and bake for 35 minutes or until a toothpick comes out clean.
6. Let cool before serving.

Dairy-free, citrus-flavored

Ingredients

- 1/2 cup olive oil
- 1 cup sugar
- 3 eggs
- Zest of 1 orange
- 1/2 cup fresh orange juice
- 1 1/2 cups all-purpose flour
- 1 tsp baking powder
- 1/4 tsp salt

Ingredient Availability

Found at Target and Publix.

Baked Apples with Cinnamon

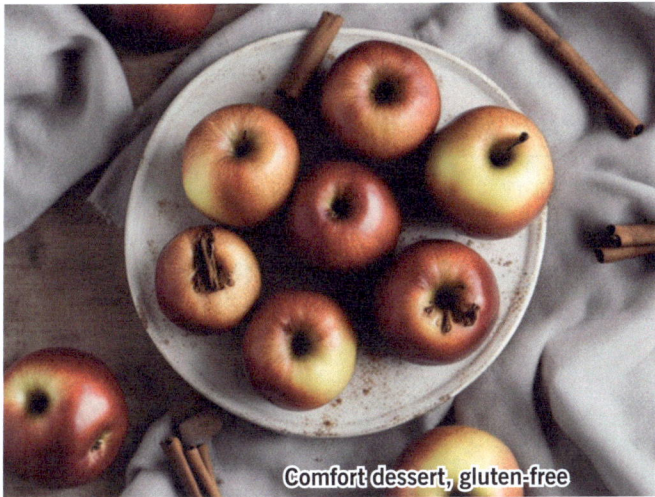

Comfort dessert, gluten-free

4 servings

Prep Time **10** min

Cook Time **25** min

Nutritional
Calories: 180 kcal
Protein: 2g
Fats: 6g
Carbs: 32g

Instructions

1. Preheat oven to 375°F (190°C).
2. Place apples in a baking dish and fill each with 1 tbsp of brown sugar and a sprinkle of cinnamon.
3. Top with walnuts and a small pat of butter.
4. Bake for 25 minutes until apples are tender.
5. Serve warm.

Ingredients

- 4 apples, cored
- 4 tbsp brown sugar
- 2 tsp cinnamon
- 1/4 cup chopped walnuts (optional)
- 2 tbsp unsalted butter

Ingredient Availability

Available at Aldi and Harris Teeter.

Dark Chocolate Covered Strawberries

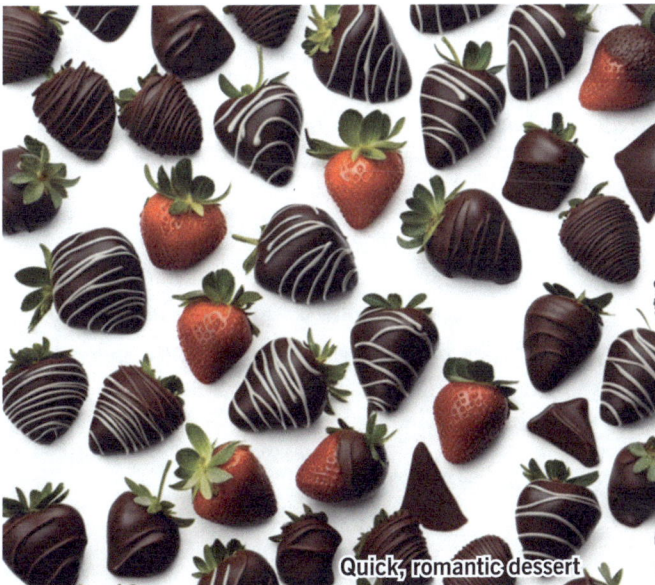

Quick, romantic dessert

4 servings

Prep Time **10** min

Cook Time **0** min

Nutritional
Calories: 150 kcal
Protein: 1g
Fats: 9g
Carbs: 18g

Instructions

1. Melt chocolate chips with coconut oil in a microwave or double boiler.
2. Dip each strawberry into the melted chocolate and place on parchment paper.
3. Let cool at room temperature or refrigerate until set.

Ingredients

- 1 cup fresh strawberries
- 1/2 cup dark chocolate chips
- 1 tsp coconut oil (optional)

Ingredient Availability

Found at Costco and Whole Foods.

Lemon Ricotta Cheesecake

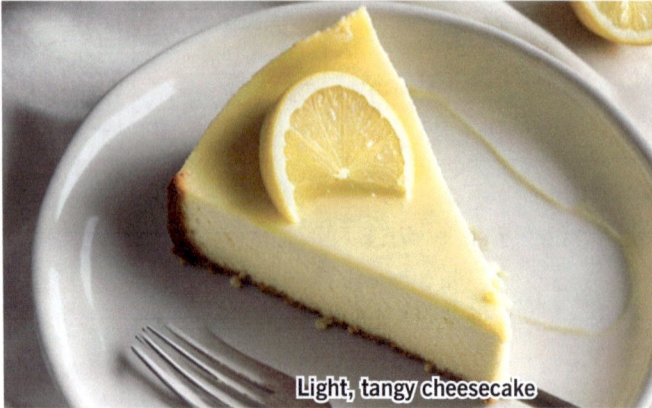

Light, tangy cheesecake

🍽 8 servings

Prep Time **20** min

Cook Time **1** h

Nutritional
Calories: 280 kcal
Protein: 8g
Fats: 15g
Carbs: 28g

Ingredients

- 1 1/2 cups ricotta cheese
- 1/2 cup cream cheese, softened
- 3/4 cup sugar
- 2 eggs
- Zest and juice of 1 lemon
- 1 tsp vanilla extract
- 1/4 cup flour

Instructions

1. Preheat oven to 350°F (175°C). Grease an 8-inch springform pan.
2. Beat ricotta and cream cheese until smooth. Add sugar and blend well.
3. Mix in eggs, one at a time. Stir in lemon zest, juice, vanilla, and flour until combined.
4. Pour mixture into the pan and bake for 1 hour.
5. Let cool before serving

Ingredient Availability

Available at Walmart and Publix.

Frozen Banana Bites with Peanut Butter

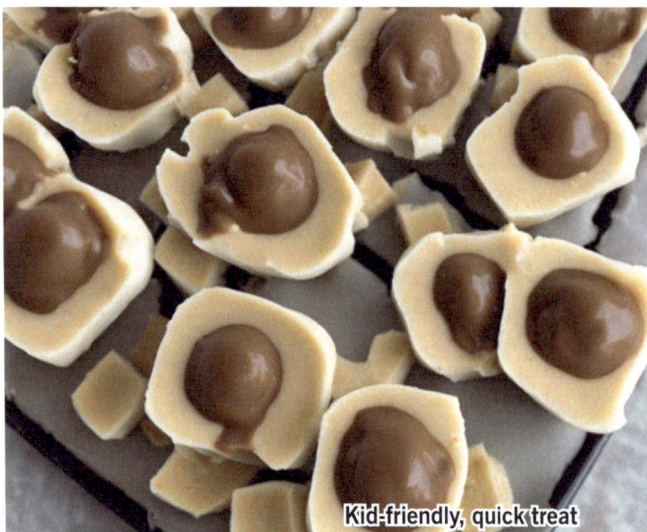

Kid-friendly, quick treat

🍽 4 servings

Prep Time **10** min

Freeze Time **1** h

Nutritional
Calories: 200 kcal
Protein: 4g
Fats: 10g
Carbs: 28g

Instructions

1. Spread peanut butter between two banana slices to make a sandwich.
2. Melt dark chocolate chips with coconut oil.
3. Dip each banana sandwich halfway in the chocolate and place on a lined tray.
4. Freeze for 1 hour before serving.

Ingredients

- 2 bananas, sliced
- 1/4 cup natural peanut butter
- 1/2 cup dark chocolate chips
- 1 tsp coconut oil (optional)

Ingredient Availability

Available at Aldi and Target.

Chia Seed Pudding with Berries

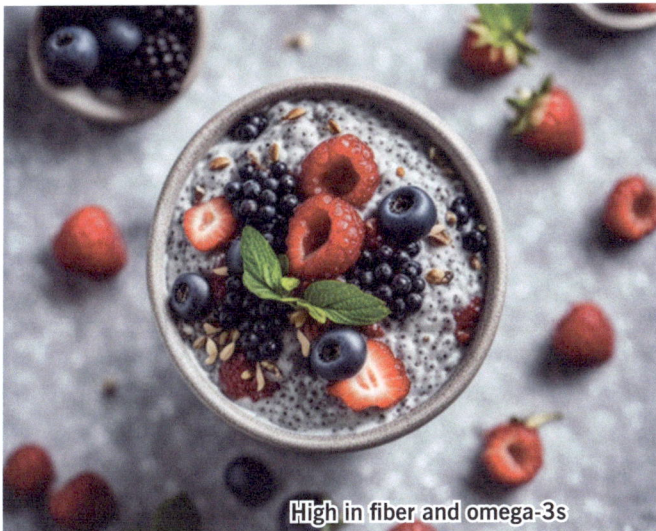

High in fiber and omega-3s

2 servings

Prep Time **5** min

Chill Time **4** h

Nutritional
Calories: 180 kcal
Protein: 4g
Fats: 8g
Carbs: 24g

Instructions

1. Combine chia seeds, almond milk, and honey in a jar. Stir well.
2. Refrigerate for 4 hours or overnight, stirring occasionally.
3. Top with mixed berries before serving.

Ingredients

- 1/4 cup chia seeds
- 1 cup almond milk
- 1 tbsp honey or maple syrup
- 1/2 cup mixed berries

Ingredient Availability

Available at Whole Foods and Costco.

Almond Flour Cookies with Dark Chocolate

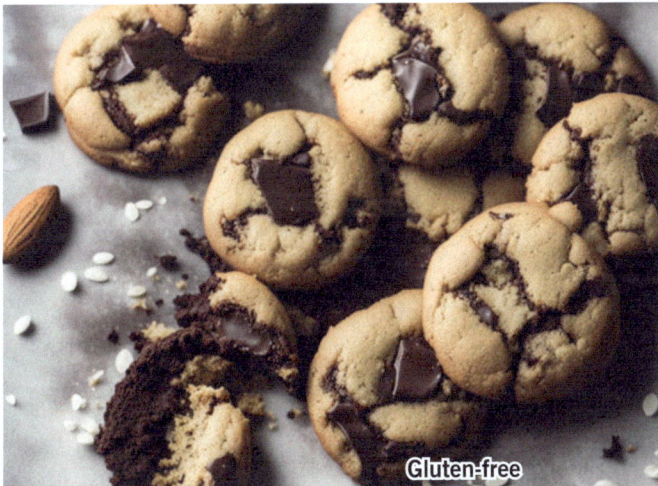

Gluten-free

12 cookies

Prep Time **10** min

Cook Time **15** min

Nutritional
Calories: 100 kcal
Protein: 2g
Fats: 8g
Carbs: 8g

Instructions

1. Preheat oven to 350°F (175°C). Line a baking sheet with parchment paper.
2. Mix all ingredients in a bowl until combined.
3. Drop spoonfuls of dough onto the sheet and flatten slightly.
4. Bake for 12-15 minutes or until golden brown.
5. Let cool on a wire rack before serving.

Ingredients

- 1 1/2 cups almond flour
- 1/4 cup dark chocolate chips
- 1/4 cup coconut oil, melted
- 1/4 cup honey
- 1 tsp vanilla extract
- 1/4 tsp baking soda
- A pinch of salt

Ingredient Availability

Available at Publix and Target.

69

Poached Pears with Spices

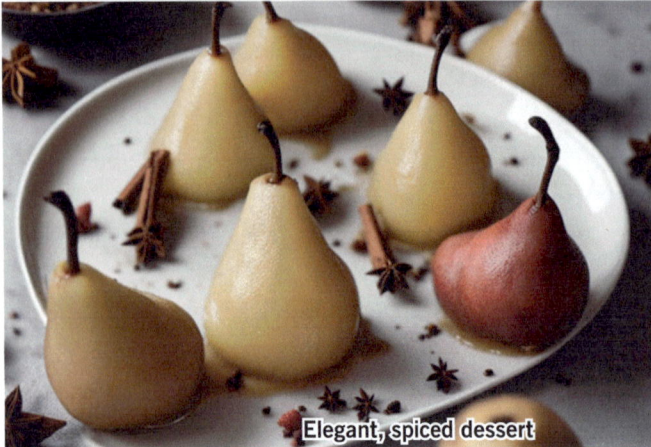

Elegant, spiced dessert

4 servings

Prep Time **10** min

Cook Time **25** min

Nutritional
Calories: 150 kcal
Protein: 1g
Fats: 0g
Carbs: 38g

Instructions

1. In a pot, bring water, honey, cinnamon, cloves, and orange zest to a simmer.
2. Add pears and poach for 20-25 minutes until tender.
3. Remove pears and reduce the syrup for 5 minutes.
4. Drizzle syrup over pears and serve warm or chilled.

Ingredients

- 4 pears, peeled and halved
- 4 cups water
- 1/2 cup honey
- 1 cinnamon stick
- 3 whole cloves
- Zest of 1 orange

Ingredient Availability

Available at Aldi and Walmart.

Pistachio and Fig Energy Bites

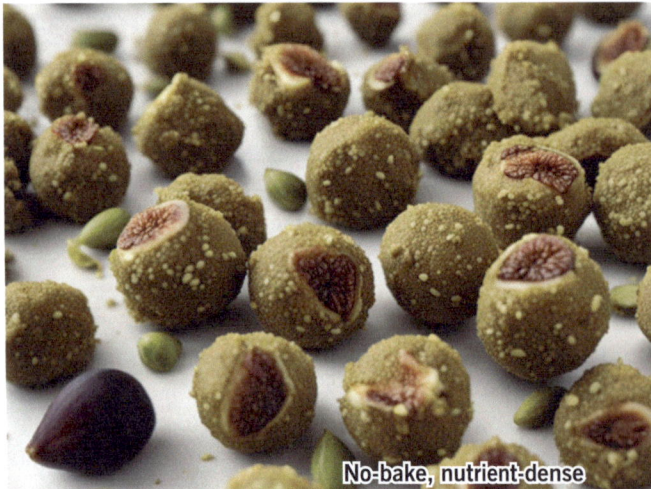

No-bake, nutrient-dense

12 bites

Prep Time **15** min

Chill Time **30** min

Nutritional
Calories: 80 kcal
Protein: 2g
Fats: 3g
Carbs: 13g

Instructions

1. Blend all ingredients in a food processor until a sticky mixture forms.
2. Roll into 12 small balls and refrigerate for 30 minutes.
3. Serve chilled.

Ingredients

- 1 cup dried figs
- 1/2 cup pistachios, shelled
- 1/2 cup almond flour
- 1 tbsp honey
- 1/2 tsp cinnamon

Ingredient Availability

Available at Whole Foods and Costco.

Chapter 9: Personalized Health Journal

The DASH diet is more than a way of eating — it's a holistic approach to nurturing long-term health and well-being. To support you on this journey, we've created a Personalized Health Journal designed to help you track progress, plan meals, and stay motivated as you embrace the DASH way of life. This journal will guide you in reflecting on your dietary habits, ensuring you stay on track and make the most of your DASH diet experience.

Simple Templates for Daily, Weekly, and Monthly Reflection

To simplify your progress tracking, the personalized health journal provides structured templates for daily, weekly, and monthly monitoring. This ensures that you can easily observe improvements, make necessary adjustments, and stay motivated to achieve your health goals.

Daily Tracking

Each day, use sections in the journal to record essential aspects of your DASH diet journey:

- **Meals:** Log your meals for breakfast, lunch, dinner, and snacks. This helps ensure you're aligning your food choices with the principles of the DASH diet, which emphasize fruits, vegetables, lean proteins, and whole grains.
- **Nutrient Intake:** Track calories, protein, fats, carbs, and sodium intake to maintain a balance. This is crucial for managing your health, especially if reducing sodium is a primary goal.
- **Energy and Mood:** Note your energy levels and mood throughout the day. This helps identify which meals provide lasting energy and overall well-being.
- **Water Intake**: Hydration is key to maintaining good health. Record your daily water intake to ensure you're drinking enough, especially when following meals rich in fiber and lean proteins.
- **Personal Notes:** Reflect on any cravings, challenges, or observations. This section allows for personal insights and adjustments as you progress through the diet.

Weekly Tracking

At the end of each week, review your progress with these sections:

- **Goals and Progress:** Set small, actionable weekly goals, such as trying a new DASH recipe, eating more vegetables, or reducing sodium intake. Reflect on your success at the week's end.
- **Weight and Measurements:** For those monitoring weight or body measurements, track changes and witness the results of your diet and lifestyle changes.
- **Well-being Reflection**: Assess your overall well-being, including energy, digestion, mood, and sleep quality. These holistic insights help fine-tune your meal plan.
- **Challenges and Adjustments:** Note any difficulties, such as eating out or managing cravings, and brainstorm solutions for the following week.

Monthly Summary

Every month, take a comprehensive look at your overall progress with the monthly summary section:

- **Achievements**: Celebrate milestones, whether it's increased energy, better digestion, or reaching a weight goal. Recognizing these successes can motivate you to continue.
- **Adjustments:** Reflect on what worked and what could be improved. For instance, consider incorporating more physical activity or trying new DASH-compliant recipes.
- **New Goals:** Set new monthly goals based on your reflections, building on the strong foundation of the DASH diet. Examples include incorporating more whole grains or reducing processed foods.

Tips for Setting and Achieving Your Health Goals

To make the most of your health journal and achieve lasting success with the DASH diet, here are some strategies:

- **Set Specific Goals**: Instead of vague objectives like "eat healthier," try concrete goals such as "include three servings of vegetables at each meal" or "limit sodium to 1,500 mg per day."
- **Stay Flexible:** Listen to your body and adjust your goals as needed. For example, if whole grains are challenging to include, try gradually incorporating different types such as quinoa or brown rice.
- **Celebrate Progress:** Small achievements lead to significant results. Whether you managed to cut back on processed foods or feel more energized, take pride in every step forward.

Adjusting Your Routine for Optimal Results

The DASH diet focuses on balance, and as you progress, it's essential to adjust your routine:

- **Energy Levels**: If energy dips, ensure you're eating enough healthy fats like avocado or olive oil.
- **Managing Cravings:** Opt for nutrient-dense snacks like carrot sticks with hummus or low-fat yogurt with fruit.
- **Weight Management:** Check portion sizes and include more leafy greens if weight loss or maintenance is a goal.

Motivation and Tips

Stay inspired with motivational quotes and practical advice sprinkled throughout the journal. These reminders will help guide you in meal prepping and making healthy choices, reinforcing the health benefits of the DASH diet.

By regularly using this personalized health journal, you'll create a clear picture of your DASH diet journey. Whether starting or continuing, tracking your progress will help you remain motivated, flexible, and ultimately successful in achieving your long-term health goals.

Chapter 10: Mastering DASH Diet Ingredients and Techniques

This chapter guides you through the essential components of the DASH Diet, from selecting and storing high-quality ingredients to mastering cooking techniques that enhance nutritional value and flavor. Whether you're a novice or an experienced cook, these tips will help you create heart-healthy, satisfying meals.

Choosing Fresh Ingredients for the DASH Diet

1. Vegetables and Fruits: Nutritional Powerhouses

- Variety is Key: Incorporate a rainbow of colors, including leafy greens, bell peppers, carrots, tomatoes, and berries. Each provides unique nutrients like potassium, magnesium, and antioxidants.

- Seasonal Selection: Choose seasonal produce for freshness, better flavor, and cost-effectiveness.

- Organic Options: If possible, prioritize organic produce for items on the «Dirty Dozen» list, such as strawberries, spinach, and kale.

2. Whole Grains

- Go for Whole: Select whole grains like quinoa, brown rice, bulgur, and whole-grain bread. Look for «100% whole grain» on packaging to ensure maximum fiber and nutrient content.

- Check Labels: Avoid products with added sugars or excessive sodium, even if labeled as whole-grain.

3. Lean Proteins

- Prioritize Lean Cuts: Opt for skinless poultry, fish, and lean cuts of beef or pork. Include plant-based proteins like lentils, beans, and tofu.

- Seafood Selection: Choose fatty fish like salmon and mackerel for heart-healthy omega-3s.

4. Low-Fat Dairy

- Healthy Choices: Use low-fat or non-fat options for milk, yogurt, and cheese to reduce saturated fat intake. Look for unsweetened varieties to avoid added sugars.

5. Healthy Fats

- Heart-Healthy Oils: Use olive oil or avocado oil for cooking and dressing.

- Nut and Seed Options: Include almonds, walnuts, flaxseeds, and chia seeds for a nutrient boost.

Proper Storage Tips for DASH-Friendly Ingredients

Vegetables and Fruits

- Refrigeration: Store most vegetables and fruits in the crisper drawer to maintain freshness.

- Freezing: Freeze fresh berries, spinach, or cooked beans in airtight bags for convenient additions to smoothies or meals.

Whole Grains

- Dry Storage: Keep grains in airtight containers in a cool, dark place to avoid moisture and pests.

- Pre-Cooked Options: Cook large batches of grains like quinoa or brown rice and store portions in the fridge or freezer for easy meal prep.

Proteins

- Refrigeration and Freezing: Store poultry, fish, and meats in the coldest part of the fridge or freeze immediately if not used within a few days. Label items with the date to ensure timely use.

- Beans and Lentils: Keep dried beans in sealed containers and canned varieties in a cool, dry pantry.

Low-Fat Dairy

- Refrigeration: Consume dairy products within their expiration dates and avoid cross-contamination by sealing containers tightly.

Herbs and Spices

- Storage: Keep dried herbs and spices in a cool, dark place to retain potency. Fresh herbs like cilantro and parsley can be stored in a jar of water in the fridge, covered loosely with a plastic bag.

Sourcing High-Quality Ingredients

Farmers' Markets

- Local Advantage: Purchase fresh, locally grown produce and dairy products. Talk to vendors to learn more about farming practices.

Grocery Stores

- Inspect Labels: Look for items labeled as «low-sodium,» «unsweetened,» or «whole grain» for DASH compliance.

- Bulk Sections: Buy grains, beans, and nuts in bulk for cost savings and reduced packaging.

Online Retailers

- Convenient Options: Use online grocers for organic produce, specialty grains, or bulk nuts and seeds.

Cooking Techniques for the DASH Diet

1. Steaming

- Retains nutrients and natural flavors of vegetables like broccoli, carrots, and zucchini.

2. Roasting

- Enhances sweetness and texture of root vegetables like sweet potatoes and beets.

3. Sautéing

- Use a small amount of olive oil to quickly cook vegetables or lean proteins while maintaining flavor.

4. Baking

- Ideal for low-fat dairy-based casseroles or lean proteins like chicken breast.

5. Grilling

- Adds a smoky flavor to vegetables, lean meats, and fish.

6. Poaching

- Gently cooks proteins like chicken or fish, keeping them tender and moist.

7. Stir-Frying

- Combines quick cooking with a variety of vegetables for a nutrient-packed dish.

Chapter 11: Product Index
for the DASH Diet

A

Alfalfa sprouts: 31

Almond butter: 5, 9, 11, 19

Almond milk: 5, 11, 15, 21, 22, 23

Almonds: 3, 4, 9, 10, 11, 15, 30, 49, 52

Apples: 5, 11, 18

Avocado: 3, 9, 10, 11, 16, 22, 24, 27, 28, 33

B

Baking powder: 17, 18, 22

Balsamic glaze: 4, 10, 34, 48

Balsamic vinegar: 12, 34, 54

Bananas: 11, 17, 22

Basil leaves: 16, 33, 34, 40, 44

Basil pesto: 28

Beets: 4, 34, 54

Berries: 3, 4, 5, 9, 10, 11, 15, 16, 18, 19, 30, 53

Black beans: 11, 32, 46

Black olives: 30

Black pepper: 12, 16, 17, 18, 19, 20, 22, 23, 24, 26, 27, 28, 29, 30, 31, 32, 33, 34, 35, 37, 38, 39, 40, 41, 42, 43, 44, 45, 46, 48, 49, 50, 51, 52, 53, 54, 55, 56, 57

Blue cheese: 26

Blueberries: 3, 9, 10, 11, 15, 16, 19

Bread: 7, 11, 12, 16, 22, 31, 33, 39, 40

Brown rice: 4, 7, 9, 10, 11, 12, 13, 37

Bulgur wheat: 53

Butter: 5, 9, 10, 11, 19, 33, 48

C

Capers: 4, 10, 12, 45, 56

Carrots: 4, 7, 11, 12, 31, 41, 51, 57

Cauliflower: 45, 48, 52

Cheddar cheese: 15, 33, 46

Cheese: 3, 4, 5, 7, 9, 10, 11, 15, 19, 20, 26, 28, 30, 33, 34, 40, 42, 44, 46, 50, 52, 54, 55

Cherry tomatoes: 4, 19, 26, 27, 28, 30, 32, 33, 38, 44, 54

Chia seeds: 3, 9, 10, 11, 17, 21

Chicken breasts: 26, 29, 37, 39, 45

Chicken broth: 45

Chives: 24, 48

Cilantro: 4, 27, 32, 46, 57

Cinnamon: 3, 5, 9, 12, 17, 19, 21, 22, 57

Coconut cream: 21

Coconut milk: 21, 35

Coconut oil: 17

Corn tortillas: 11

Cottage cheese: 3, 9, 10, 11, 20

Cream cheese: 11, 20

Croutons: 26

Cucumber: 3, 4, 5, 7, 9, 10, 11, 13, 24, 26, 27, 30, 31, 32, 35, 37, 51

Cumin: 12, 32, 46, 52, 57

D

Dijon mustard: 26, 39, 43

Dill: 3, 5, 9, 10, 11, 12, 18, 20, 24, 29, 50, 54

Dried cranberries: 4, 30, 53

Dried oregano: 19, 37, 42, 44, 50

E

Edamame: 5, 9, 10, 11, 35, 37

Eggs: 3, 10, 11, 13, 15, 17, 22, 23, 24

Enchilada sauce: 46

F

Firm tofu: 45

Flour: 5

G

Garlic cloves: 12, 34

Garlic powder: 40, 45, 55, 57

Goat cheese: 4, 34, 54

Greek yogurt: 3, 5, 9, 10, 12, 16, 24, 26, 29

Green beans: 4, 11, 49

Green bell pepper: 17

Greens: 7, 11, 13, 27, 29

Ground turkey: 4, 11, 40, 42

H

Heavy cream: 11, 48

Honey: 3, 4, 5, 9, 10, 15, 16, 17, 18, 19, 20, 21, 22, 23, 35, 37, 43

Hummus: 3, 4, 5, 9, 10, 12, 28, 31

I

Ice cubes: 23

J

Jalapeño: 46

Jasmine rice: 45

L

Leeks: 45

Lemon juice: 26, 27, 29, 30, 32, 33, 37, 39, 43, 45, 49, 56

Lemon zest: 24, 49

Lentils: 11, 26, 54

Lime juice: 32, 46

M

Mahi-mahi fillets: 46

Mango: 3, 4, 5, 9, 10, 11, 21, 29, 46

Maple syrup: 19, 21, 22

Milk: 5, 7, 11, 15, 17, 18, 21, 22, 23, 35

Mint: 3, 5, 9, 11, 13, 20, 24, 32

Mozzarella cheese: 40

Mushrooms: 4, 15, 44, 52

Mustard: 4, 9, 26, 39, 43

O

Oats: 3, 9, 11, 12, 15, 17, 21, 22

P

Olive oil: 5, 7, 11, 13, 15, 16, 17, 18, 19, 22, 23, 24, 26, 27, 30, 32, 33, 34, 35, 37, 38, 39, 40, 41, 42, 43, 44, 45, 46, 48, 49, 50, 51, 52, 53, 54, 55, 56, 57

P

Paprika: 12, 18, 39, 45, 50, 53, 57

Parmesan cheese: 26, 28, 40, 42, 55

Parsley: 11, 17, 18, 24, 26, 32, 43, 44, 45, 49, 51, 54, 57

Pineapple: 3, 5, 9, 10, 11, 20

Portobello mushrooms: 44

Q

Quinoa: 3, 4, 7, 9, 10, 11, 12, 13, 19, 27, 34, 44, 49

R

Red bell pepper: 17, 27, 31, 38, 39

Red cabbage: 11, 35, 37

Red onion: 17, 18, 26, 29, 30, 32, 39, 46, 51, 54

Red wine vinegar: 51, 54, 56

Rice vinegar: 35, 37

Ricotta cheese: 5, 11

Rosemary: 4, 9, 10, 12, 39, 41, 57

Russet potatoes: 50

S

Salt: 9, 12, 15, 16, 17, 18, 19, 20, 22, 23, 24, 26, 27, 28, 29, 30, 31, 32, 33, 34, 35, 37, 38, 39, 40, 41, 42, 43, 44, 45, 46, 48, 49, 50, 51, 52, 53, 54, 55, 56, 57

Sesame seeds: 35, 37, 41

Soy sauce: 35, 37, 38, 41

Spaghetti squash: 4, 9, 10, 42

Spinach: 3, 4, 9, 10, 11, 13, 15, 19, 23, 28, 31, 33, 35, 52

Sun-dried tomatoes: 40

Sweet potatoes: 11, 18, 46, 53

T

Thyme: 4, 9, 10, 12, 39, 41, 51, 55

Tomato: 3, 4, 5, 7, 9, 10, 11, 12, 16, 19, 22, 26, 27, 28, 30, 32, 33, 34, 35, 38, 40, 44, 51, 54, 55, 56

Tuna: 3, 9, 10, 11, 29

U

Unsweetened applesauce: 18

V

Vegetable broth: 12, 49, 53, 54

W

Walnuts: 3, 5, 9, 10, 16, 22, 34

Water: 5, 8, 9, 10, 13, 15, 19, 21, 23, 26, 29

White vinegar: 23

Wraps: 3, 9, 10, 12, 28, 31

Z

Zucchini: 3, 4, 5, 9, 10, 11, 12, 28, 39, 44, 50, 55

Conclusion

As you conclude your journey through the DASH Diet Cookbook for Beginners, it's essential to reflect on the progress you've made and the tools you've acquired to maintain a heart-healthy lifestyle. The DASH (Dietary Approaches to Stop Hypertension) diet is more than a temporary eating plan; it's a sustainable approach to nutrition that emphasizes balance, variety, and moderation.

Final Words of Encouragement

Embarking on the DASH diet is a commendable step toward improving your health. Transitioning to a new dietary pattern can be challenging, but remember that each small change contributes to your overall well-being. Celebrate your successes, no matter how minor they may seem, and view setbacks as opportunities to learn and grow. Consistency is key; over time, these healthier choices will become second nature.

Additional Resources for Continued Success

To support your ongoing journey with the DASH diet, consider exploring the following reputable resources:

- **National Heart, Lung, and Blood Institute (NHLBI):** The NHLBI offers comprehensive guides and resources on the DASH eating plan, including meal planning tools and tips for reducing sodium intake.
- **American Heart Association (AHA):** The AHA provides information on heart-healthy eating patterns, including the DASH diet, along with recipes and dietary recommendations.
- **Mayo Clinic:** The Mayo Clinic offers detailed articles on the DASH diet, including sample menus and insights into its health benefits.
- **Harvard T.H. Chan School of Public Health:** This resource provides an in-depth review of the DASH diet, discussing its components and health implications.

These resources can provide additional guidance, recipes, and support as you continue to embrace the DASH diet.

Join the DASH Diet Community Online

Connecting with others who are following the DASH diet can offer motivation, support, and shared experiences. Consider joining online communities and forums where members exchange tips, recipes, and encouragement. Engaging with a community can provide a sense of accountability and make your journey more enjoyable.

Remember, adopting the DASH diet is a positive step toward a healthier lifestyle. With the knowledge and resources provided in this cookbook, along with the support of the broader community, you're well-equipped to continue making heart-healthy choices that will benefit you for years to come.

Made in United States
Troutdale, OR
05/04/2025

31098873R00044